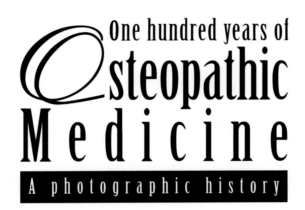

One hundred years of

Osteopathic Medicine

A photographic history

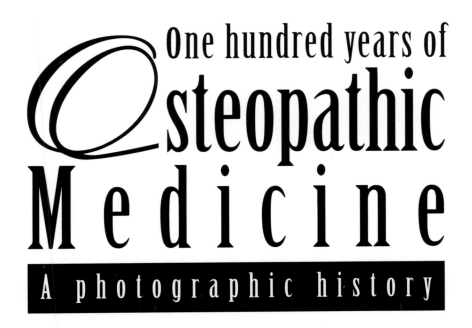

One hundred years of Osteopathic Medicine

A photographic history

with commentary by

Warren K. Klofkorn and J. Lynne Dodson

GP **Greenwich Press**
Greenwich Connecticut

Greenwich Press
Greenwich Office Park #6
Greenwich, CT 06830

ISBN: 1-57013-036-1

Publisher: Corey Kupersmith, RPh
Editorial Director: Lois Gandt
Art Director: Jill Ruscoll

Printed in Hong Kong

Introduction

In 1889 Benjamin Harrison was inaugurated as the 23rd president of the United States. Four Western states—North and South Dakota, Montana, and Washington—entered the Union. We were a growing boisterous, confident nation, recovering admirably from the ravages of the Civil War 25 years earlier.

That war had brought significant changes to aspects of allopathic medicine, particularly surgery. Creation of the field hospital system, a more conservative view toward limb amputations, and the use of antiseptic wound care were among them. Nevertheless, to many sufferers of common chronic and acute diseases, traditional medicine seemed to offer little relief. Many physicians were slow to experiment or to embrace the results of others' experiments, slow to change even in the face of medical evidence. Not surprisingly, perhaps, alternative medicines flourished, especially in the individualist territories west of the Mississippi River.

One of these alternatives was osteopathic medicine, formulated by Dr Andrew Taylor Still in 1889. Within three years he would found a school in Kirksville, Missouri, to teach others his techniques. One hundred years later, 15 schools in the United States continue to train osteopathic practitioners and conduct research to advance the field.

Throughout this history, the camera was there. Included in this volume are photographs of Still's hands-on teaching methods and the first graduating class, which posed solemnly with Dr Still and his teaching skeleton, "Columbus." Today's students are caught by the camera as they work in their communities, classrooms, and laboratories.

This photographic history offers unprecedented documentation of a significant medical development of our century.

Contents

the
Beginnings

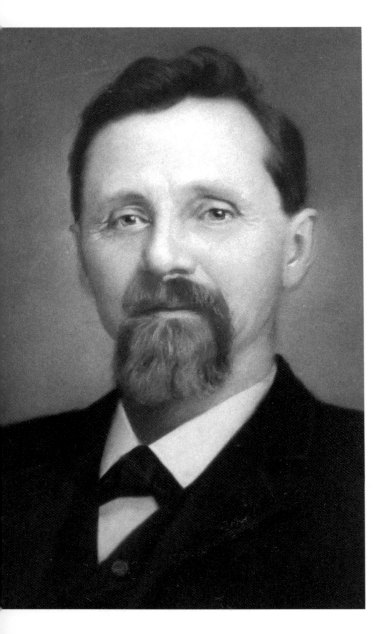

Dr Andrew Taylor Still realized a reformation of medical thought and practice when in 1889 he "flung to the breeze the banner of osteopathy." Against the tide of popular mediocrity and resistance to change, Dr Still challenged the medical and scientific establishment of his day, holding fast to his convictions in the face of social pressures and intellectual ostracism. The discrepancy between the primitive state of medical knowledge and the hubris of the physicians of the day set the stage for the drama that unfolded as Dr Still first formulated and then advanced his new model of medicine—osteopathy.

A. T. Still always maintained that osteopathy came to him as an original and unprecedented idea. However, osteopathy arrived on the scene during a period when many alternative systems of medicine flourished. Some of these approaches continued to attract adherents over subsequent decades. Homeopathy retains some popularity even today; others, such as hydrotherapy and mechanotherapy, popularized by the Zander Institute, lapsed into obscurity.

Left: *A portrait of Andrew Taylor Still created by Floyd W. Horton, circa 1895.*

Right: *The log cabin in which A. T. Still was born, shown adjacent to the Still National Osteopathic Museum, Kirksville, Missouri, circa 1985.*

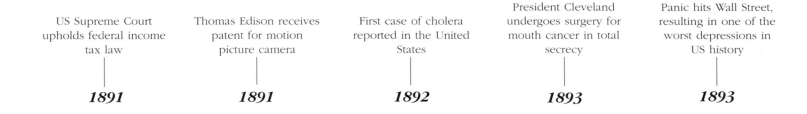

US Supreme Court upholds federal income tax law	Thomas Edison receives patent for motion picture camera	First case of cholera reported in the United States	President Cleveland undergoes surgery for mouth cancer in total secrecy	Panic hits Wall Street, resulting in one of the worst depressions in US history
1891	*1891*	*1892*	*1893*	*1893*

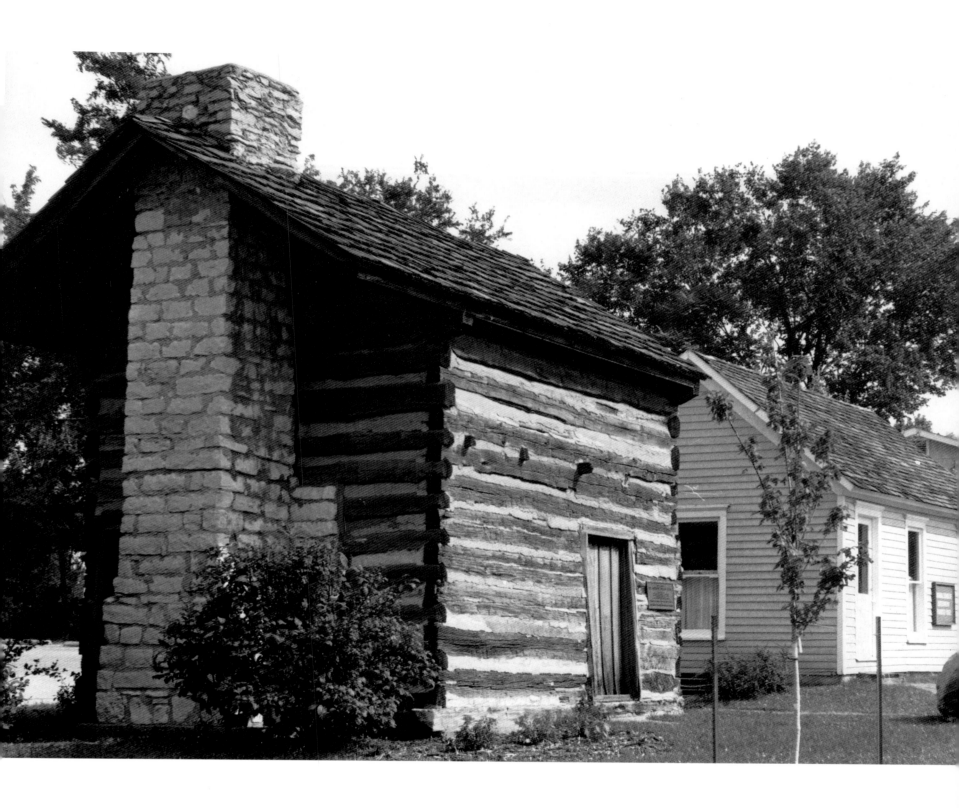

Fire destroys almost all of the buildings in Chicago's Columbian Exposition, with $2 million in damage

1894

X-rays are used in the United States for the first time, for cancer therapy

1896

First modern Olympic Games are held in Athens, Greece, with the United States winning nine of 12 events

1896

Gold is discovered in the Klondike and the Canadian Gold Rush begins

1896

The battleship *Maine* explodes in Havana Harbor, precipitating war between the United States and Spain

1898

Above: *A. T. Still's handwritten definition of osteopathy. The original is written on fragile, wood-pulp paper in dull pencil.*

Right: *The son of a Methodist minister, A. T. Still considered the human body to be a divinely ordained creation.*

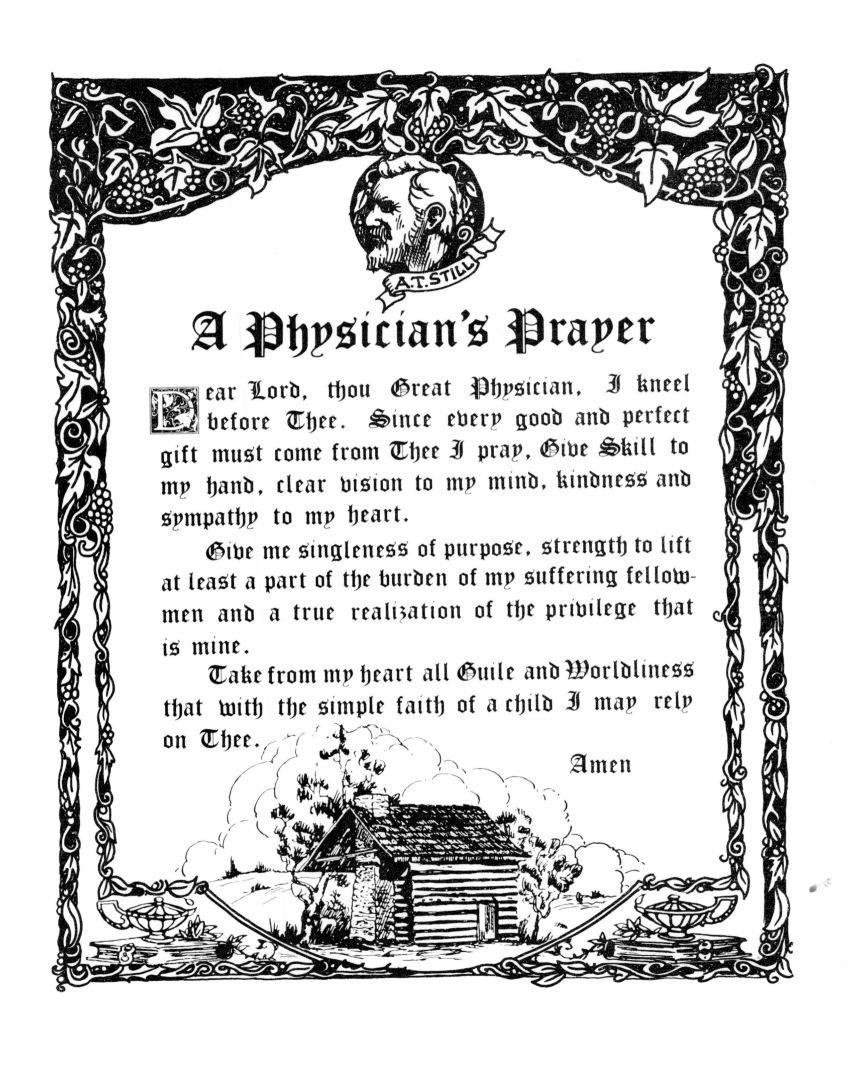

A Physician's Prayer

Dear Lord, thou Great Physician, I kneel before Thee. Since every good and perfect gift must come from Thee I pray, Give Skill to my hand, clear vision to my mind, kindness and sympathy to my heart.

Give me singleness of purpose, strength to lift at least a part of the burden of my suffering fellow-men and a true realization of the privilege that is mine.

Take from my heart all Guile and Worldliness that with the simple faith of a child I may rely on Thee.

Amen

A. T. Still built a thriving practice in his new science of osteopathy, giving new hope to patients who often had found none with practitioners of traditional medicine. In 1892 he established the American School of Osteopathy, the first school of osteopathy, in the primitive setting of a two-room, frame building on the outskirts of Kirksville, Missouri. The furnishings of that first school were sparse, but even so the classes of students crowded the tiny building. One of Dr Still's few teaching aids in those early days was a skeleton used to teach anatomy.

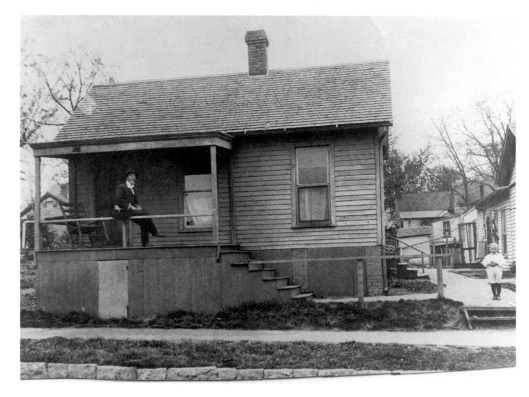

Above: *Dr Still posed at the building that housed the first school of osteopathy. The main building contains two rooms plus an addition (not shown) in the rear.*

Right: *Dr Still's roll-top desk, as currently exhibited in the first school building on the campus of the Kirksville College of Osteopathic Medicine.*

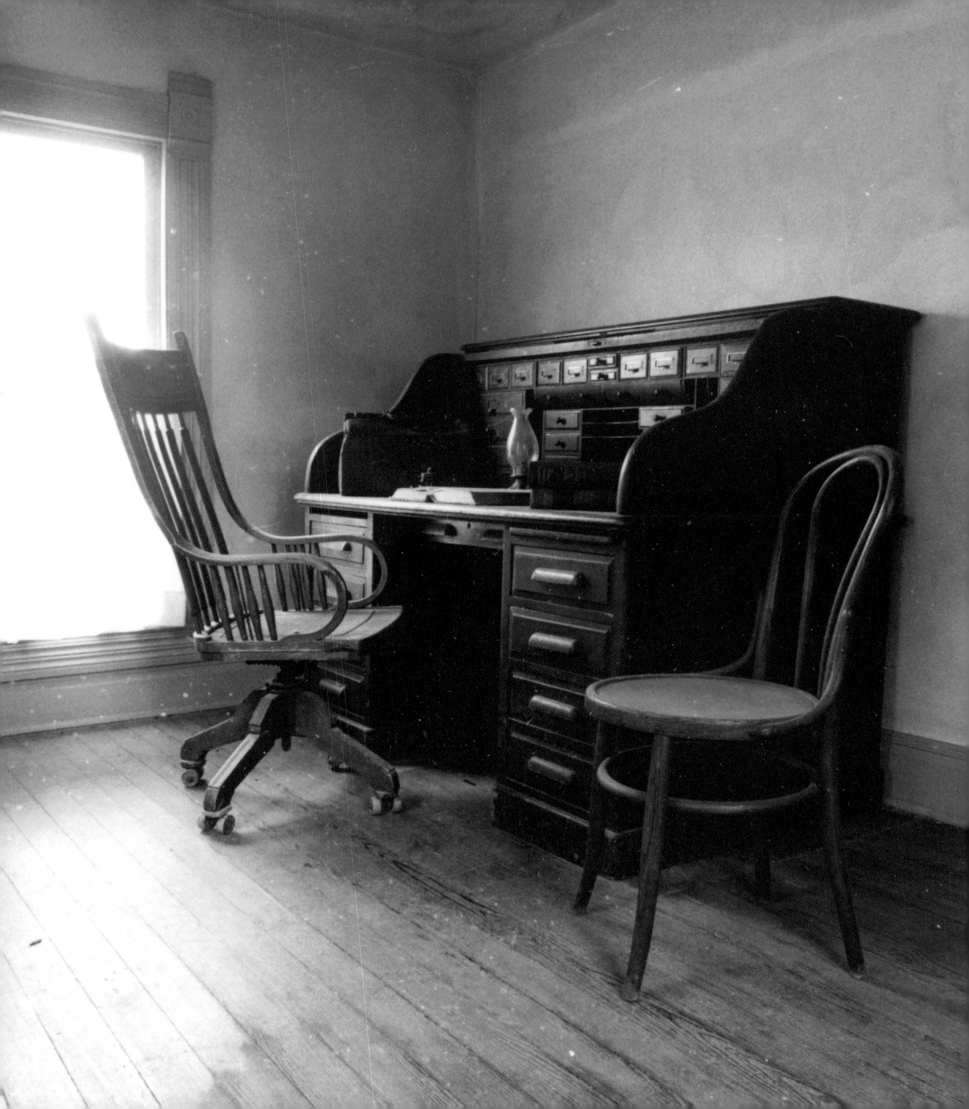

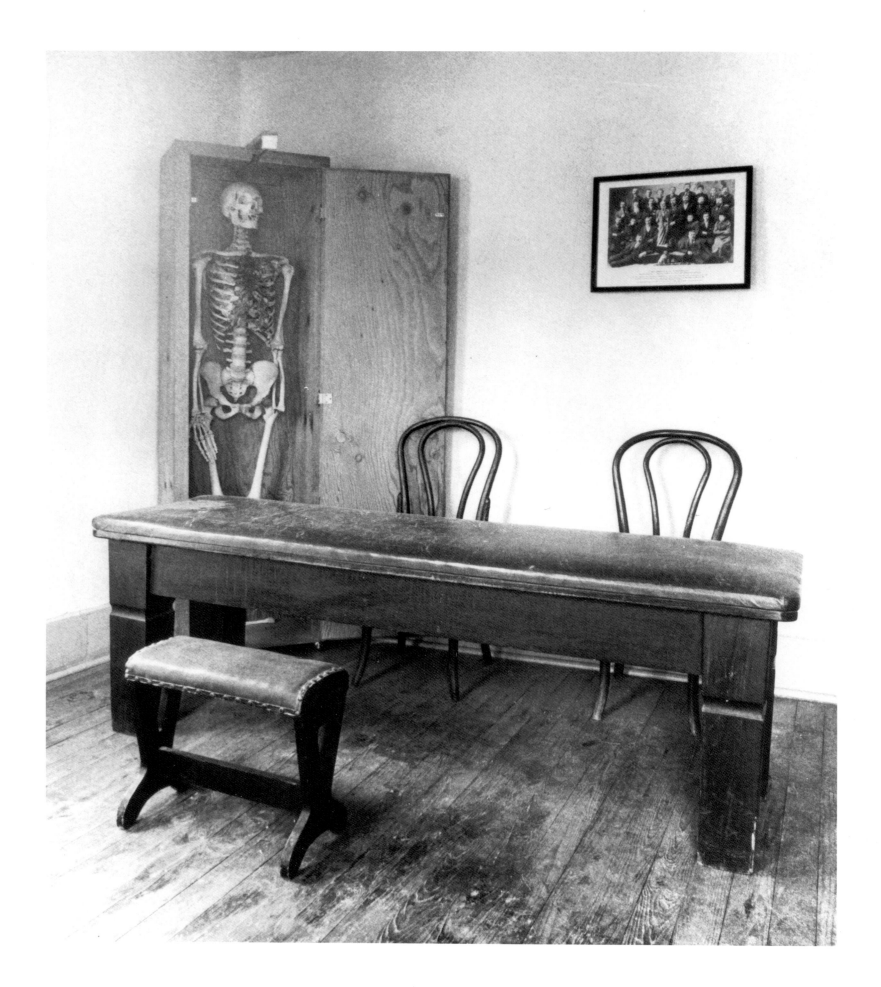

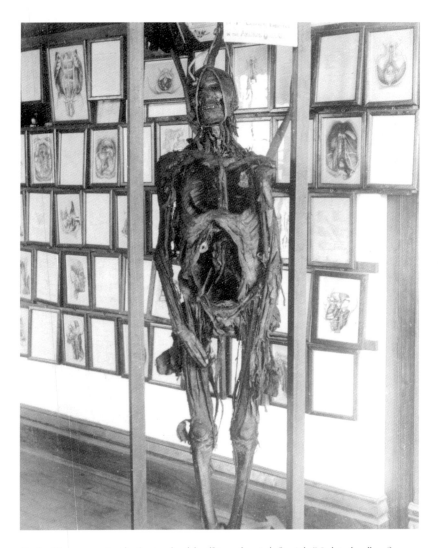

Left: *Classroom in the first school building, furnished with "Columbus" and an early osteopathic treatment table.*

Above: *Anatomy was central to the teaching of osteopathy from the very beginning. The first cadaver at the American School of Osteopathy was named "Mike."*

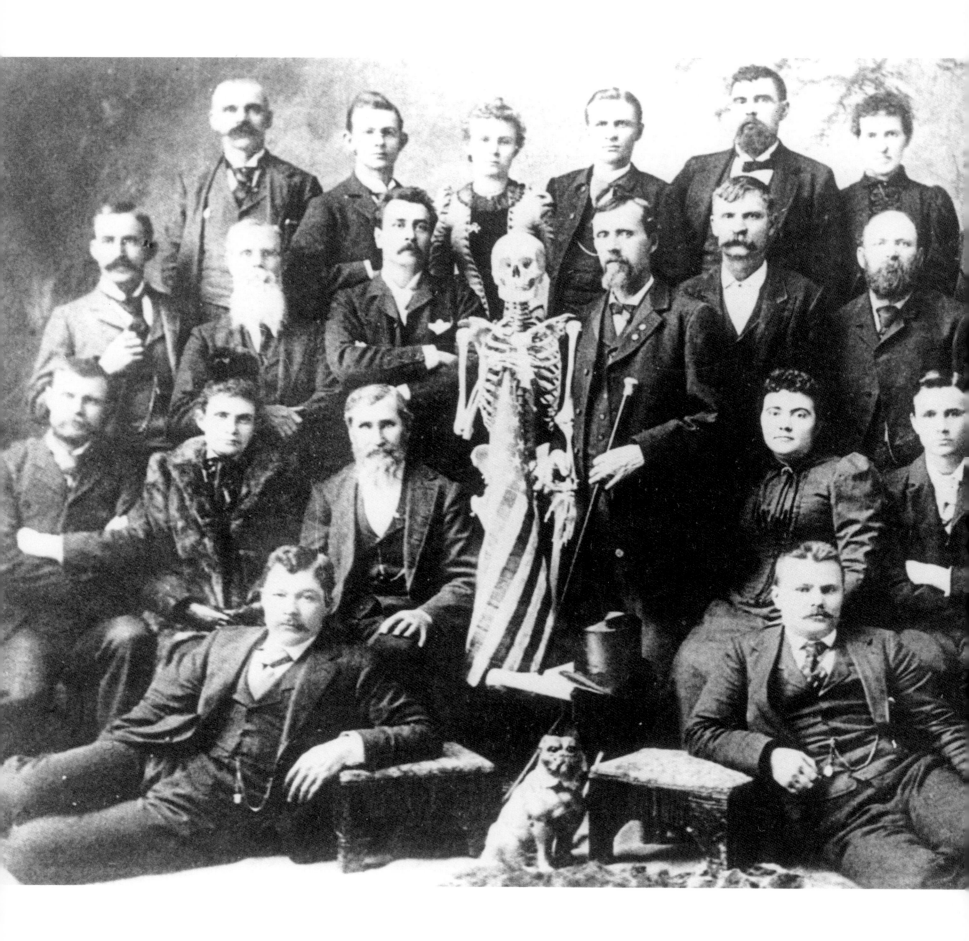

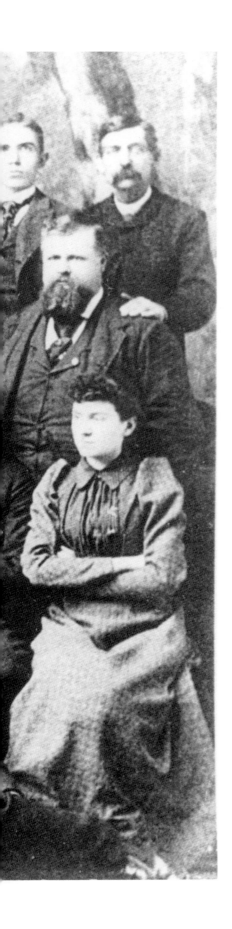

American School of Osteopathy

Know all men by these presents, that
William Smith, M.D.
having attended a full course of Lectures on, and
Demonstrations of Osteopathy, and having, after due
examination, been found fully qualified to practise the
Art in all its branches, is hereby conferred by me
with the title
Diplomate in Osteopathy.

Given at Kirksville, Missouri
this, the 15th day of February 1893

A.J. Still
President

Left: *The first class in osteopathy, 1892-93, with Dr Still in the center, next to "Columbus." The group included five women and five members of the Still family.*

Above: *The first diploma awarded by the American School of Osteopathy. It was given to William Smith, MD, who served as the school's first teacher of anatomy.*

The rapid growth of the American School of Osteopathy necessitated construction that must have seemed nearly continuous to the people of Kirksville. Within 2 years of commencing instruction, Dr Still and his faculty built the A. T. Still Infirmary—a building that housed clinic facilities, classrooms, an anatomy laboratory, and an office for Dr Still. By 1897, two separate additions had been added to the Infirmary. A maternity hospital was added in 1895, and then converted for use as the A. T. Still Surgical Sanitorium in 1898. Also in 1898 a reservoir for the facilities with its own steam-powered pumping station was added half a mile west of the complex.

Before the end of the first decade of the ASO, the science of osteopathy was spreading across the country. New schools were established rapidly in widely separated locations such as Des Moines, Iowa, Chicago, Philadelphia, and Anaheim, California.

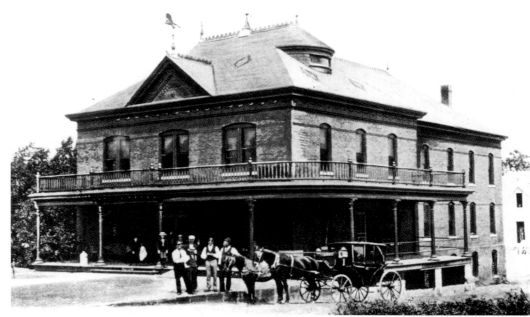

Above: *This colonial-style structure housed the A. T. Still Infirmary, built in 1894.*

Right: *Warren Hamilton, DO, in the business office of the Kirksville school, circa 1899.*

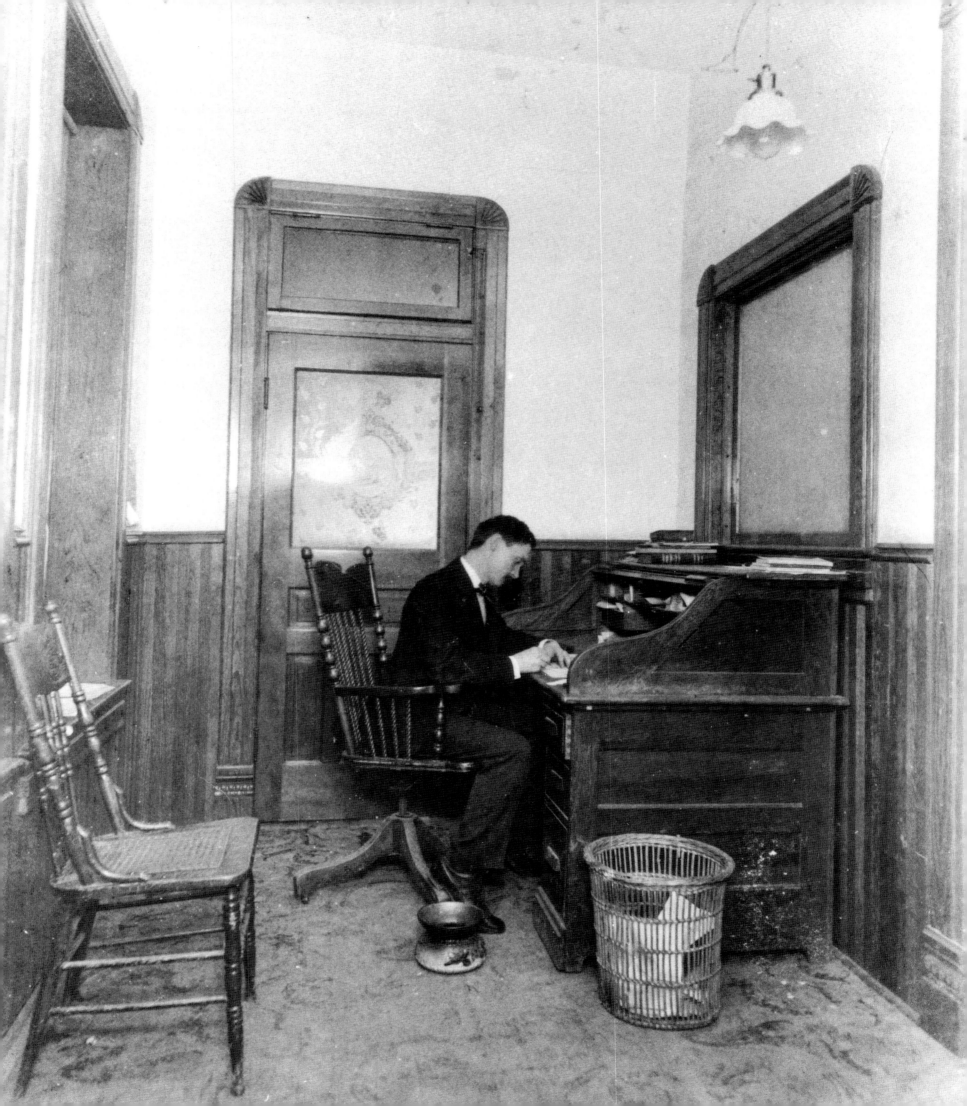

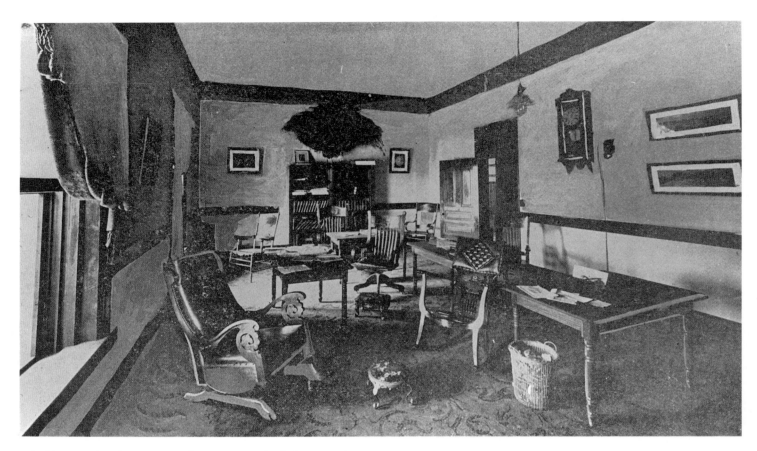

The library and reading room at the American School of Osteopathy.

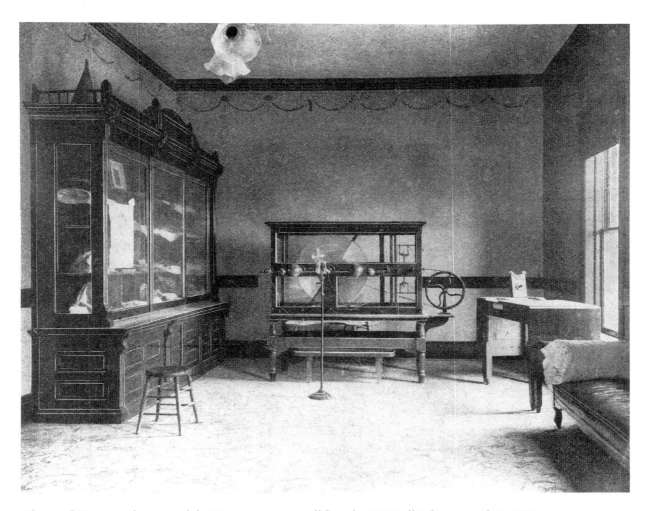

The second X-ray machine west of the Mississippi was installed at the A. T. Still Infirmary early in 1899.

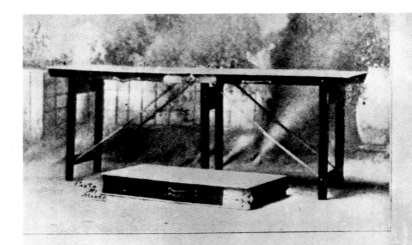

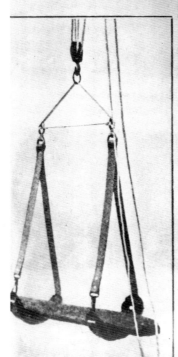

A variety of osteopathic treatment aids, including this table and swing, were produced over the years. A table similar to this one is displayed at the Still National Osteopathic Museum.

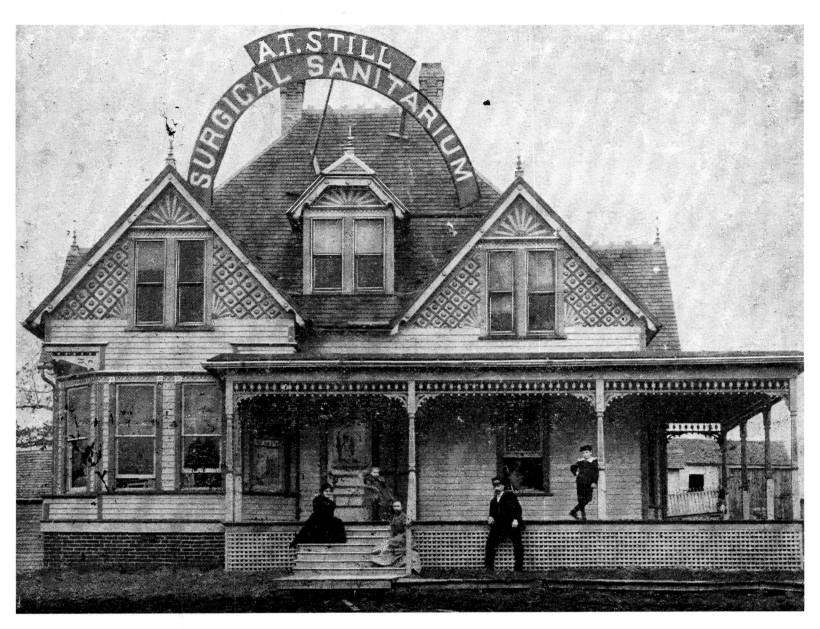

The A. T. Still Surgical Sanitarium served the school from 1898 until 1905, when a new hospital was opened. This building was destroyed by fire in 1921.

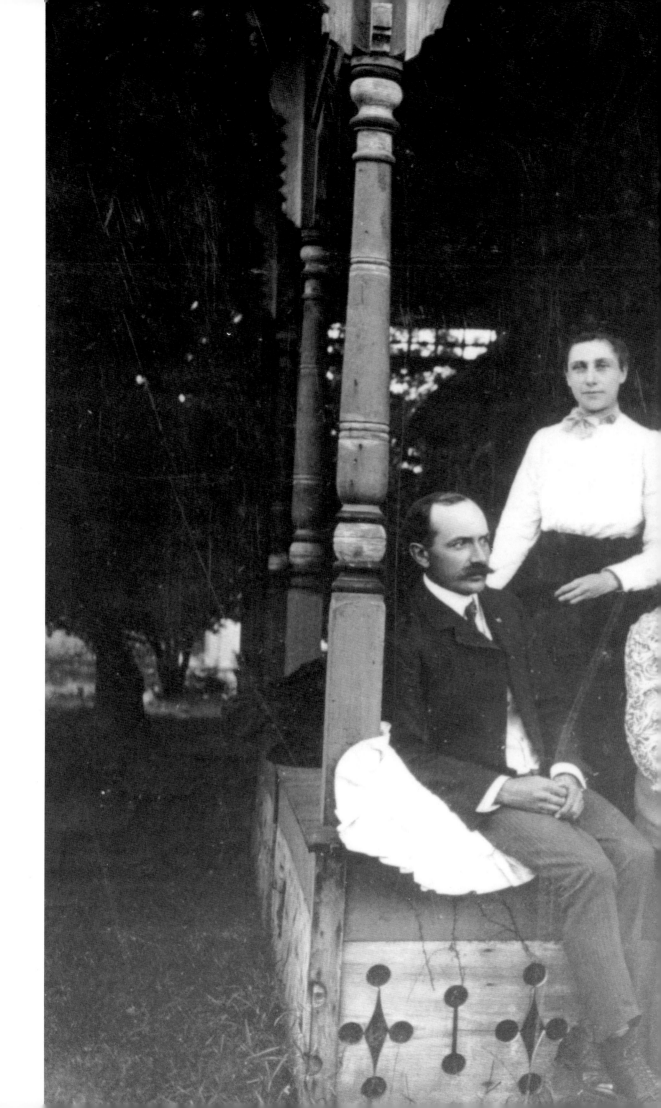

Graduates of the American School of Osteopathy relocated in many parts of the country. This photograph was taken at the West Infirmary of Osteopathy in Iowa around the turn of the century.

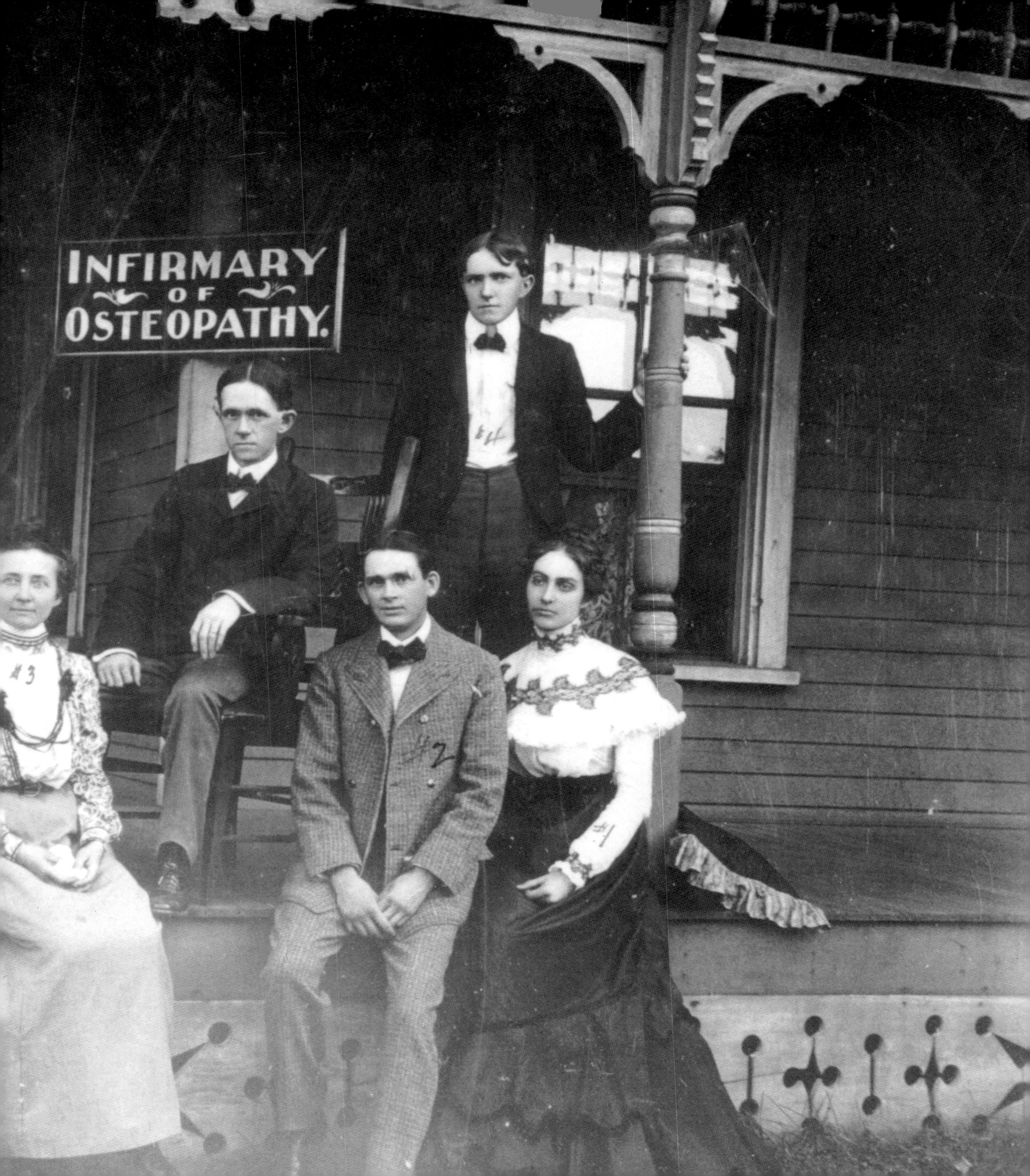
INFIRMARY
OF
OSTEOPATHY.

One distinctive feature of osteopathic medicine even in its infancy was that women were allowed to enroll as students for the DO degree, in contrast to the practice of American allopathic schools of the time, which universally prohibited women from matriculation. In fact, women were members of the very first graduating class at the ASO, and soon occupied faculty positions.

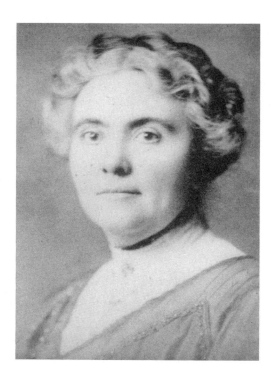

Jeanette Bolles, BA, DO, was a member of the first graduating class of the American School of Osteopathy and later taught anatomy at the school.

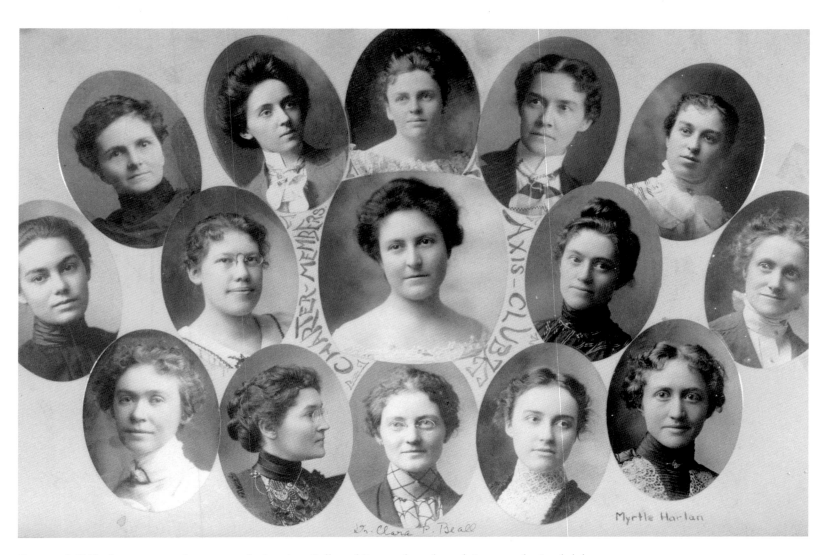

By around 1898, there were enough women at the American College of Osteopathy to form their own professional club.

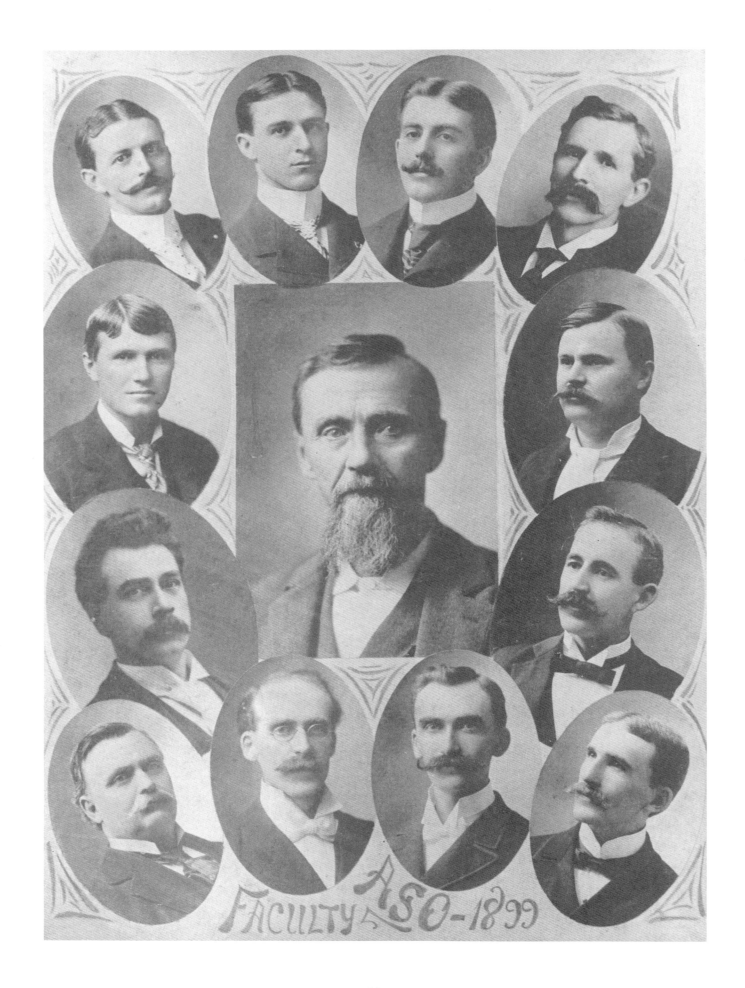

32

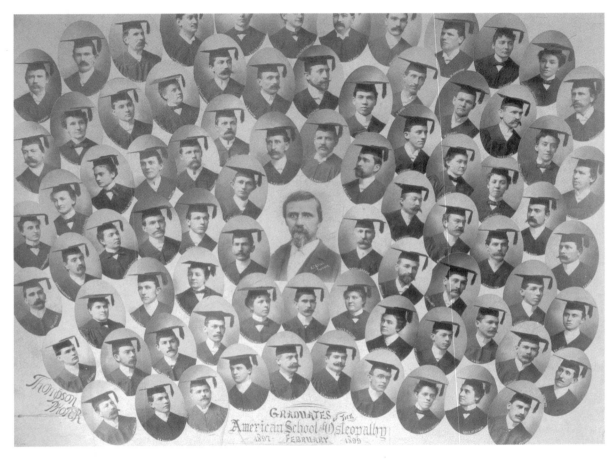

Left: *Dr Still and the Kirksville faculty in 1899.*

Above: *The class of 1899 included two future presidents, a trustee, and an assistant secretary, all of the American Osteopathic Association, and the founder of* Popular Osteopath, *the precursor to the* AOA Journal.

Faced with increasingly organized and vocal opposition from the allopathic medical profession, Daniel B. Macauley, DO, and other osteopaths situated in and around Kirksville organized the American Association for the Advancement of Osteopathy, ratifying its constitution in April of 1897. Four years later, when the AAAO had its annual convention in Kirksville, the association changed its name to the American Osteopathic Association.

The purpose of the new organization was stated in the preamble to the constitution of the AAAO:

"In order to conserve, consolidate, and propagate the therapeutic science and practice of Osteopathy and to secure for it a compact and complete organization, a commanding recognition, a pervasive influence and a professional *esprit de corps* among its students and practitioners, we, the friends and followers of Osteopathy, upon conditions to be hereafter specified, realizing the significance and importance of this science in the march and movement of the world's thought, and in its relation to all other therapeutic arts and agencies, and the well-being of the sick and suffering of our common humanity, do hereby resolve to organize and constitute ourselves into a formal Osteopathic Society."

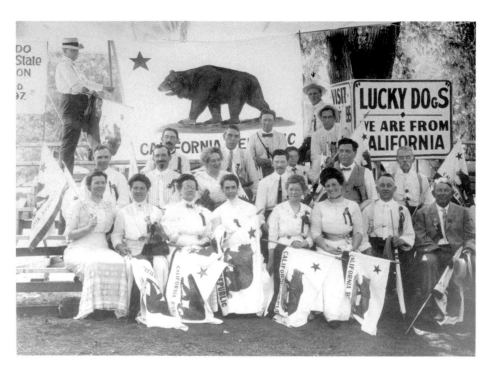

Above: *The California delegation to an American Osteopathic Association convention early in this century.*

Right: *The first five presidents of the American Osteopathic Association.*

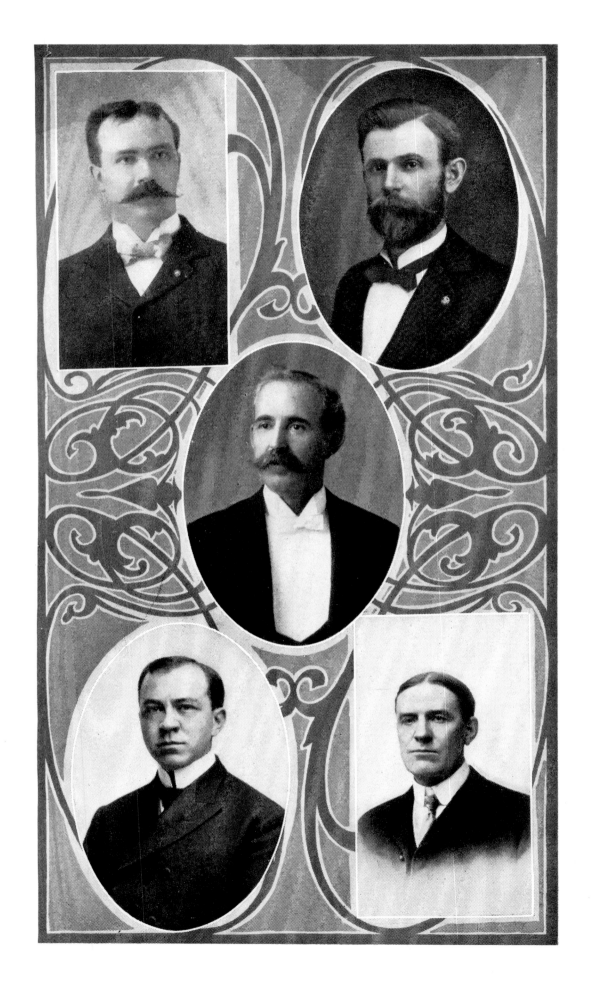

gaining Ground

By 1900 the American School of Osteopathy had more than 700 graduates, most of whom established practices outside of Missouri. Several of these graduates also opened their own schools of osteopathy in Kansas City, Los Angeles, and Minneapolis. Within a few years more than a dozen schools were teaching osteopathic principles and techniques. These programs typically followed the format of the American School of Osteopathy, charging up to $500 for a 20-month course of study.

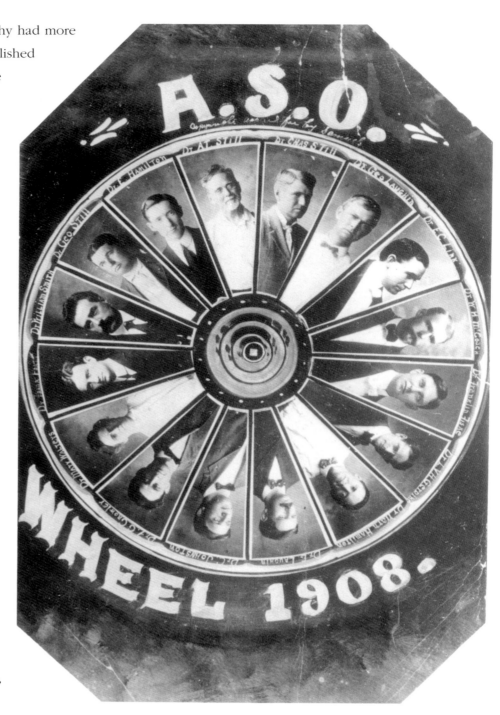

In 1908 the faculty of the American School of Osteopathy included three members of the Still family and one woman, Dr Mary Walters.

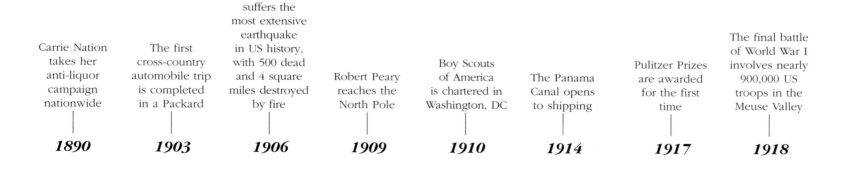

Carrie Nation takes her anti-liquor campaign nationwide	The first cross-country automobile trip is completed in a Packard	San Francisco suffers the most extensive earthquake in US history, with 500 dead and 4 square miles destroyed by fire	Robert Peary reaches the North Pole	Boy Scouts of America is chartered in Washington, DC	The Panama Canal opens to shipping	Pulitzer Prizes are awarded for the first time	The final battle of World War I involves nearly 900,000 US troops in the Meuse Valley
1890	*1903*	*1906*	*1909*	*1910*	*1914*	*1917*	*1918*

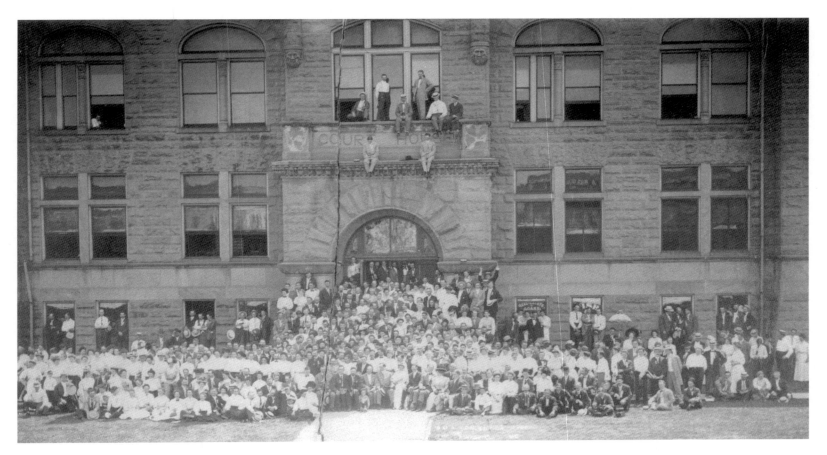

In August 1908, osteopathic physicians from around the world posed on the steps of the county courthouse in Kirksville, Missouri, during the celebration for the 80th birthday of A. T. Still.

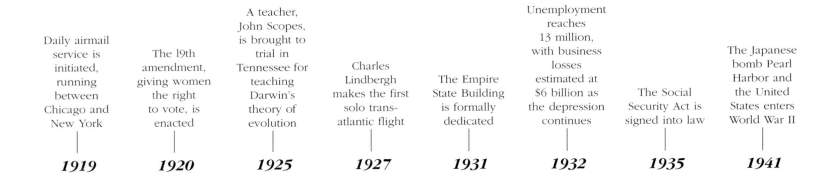

Daily airmail service is initiated, running between Chicago and New York

1919

The 19th amendment, giving women the right to vote, is enacted

1920

A teacher, John Scopes, is brought to trial in Tennessee for teaching Darwin's theory of evolution

1925

Charles Lindbergh makes the first solo trans-atlantic flight

1927

The Empire State Building is formally dedicated

1931

Unemployment reaches 13 million, with business losses estimated at $6 billion as the depression continues

1932

The Social Security Act is signed into law

1935

The Japanese bomb Pearl Harbor and the United States enters World War II

1941

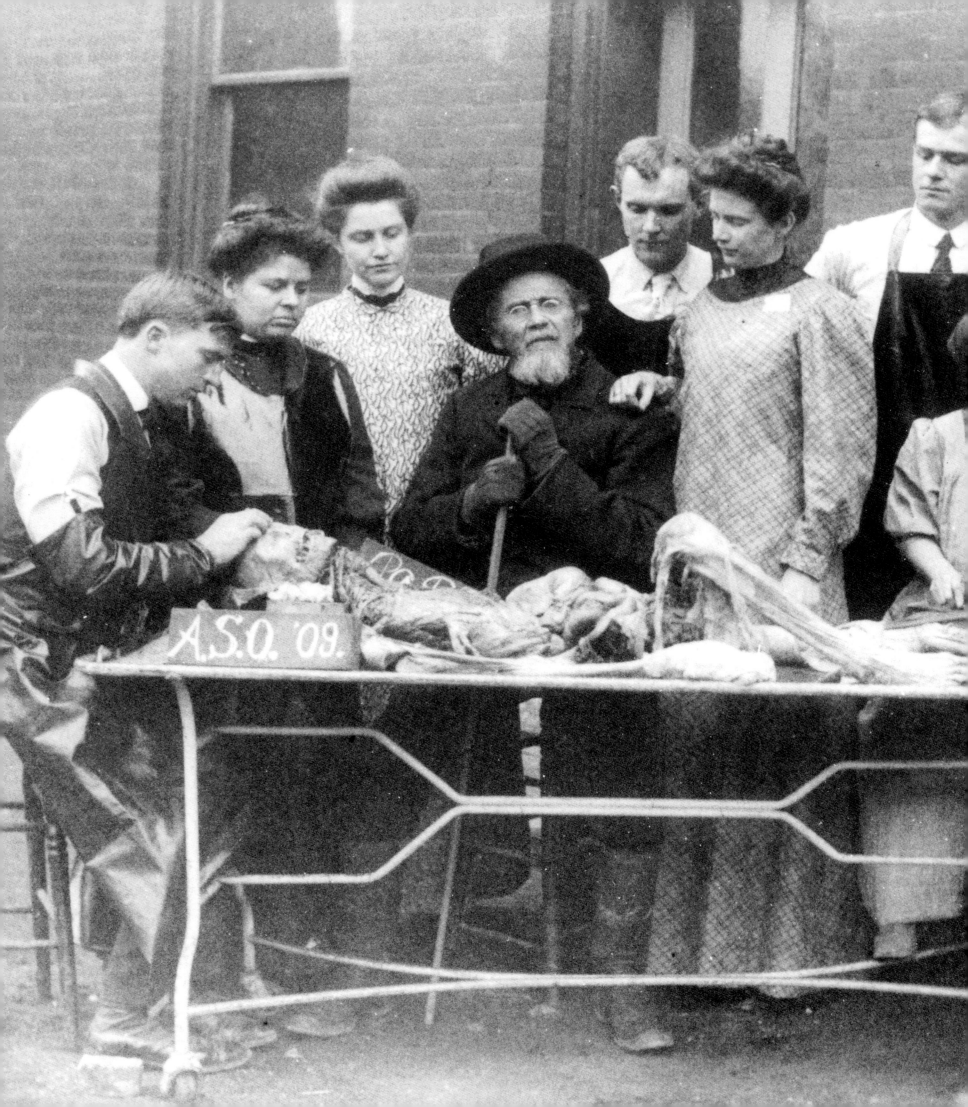

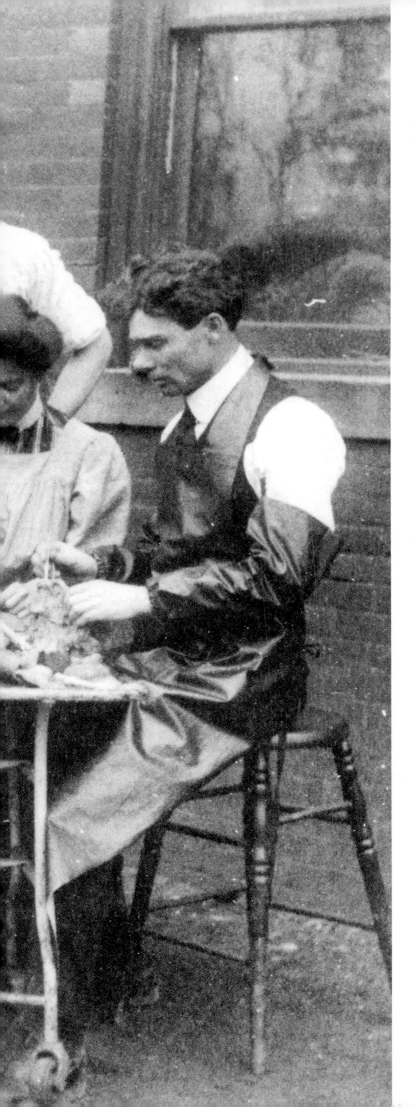

The 1909 anatomy class of the American School of Osteopathy. The dissection classes routinely posed for group photographs with their cadaver subjects—often positioning the cadavers in humorous counterpoint to what otherwise might be taken as a grim scene.

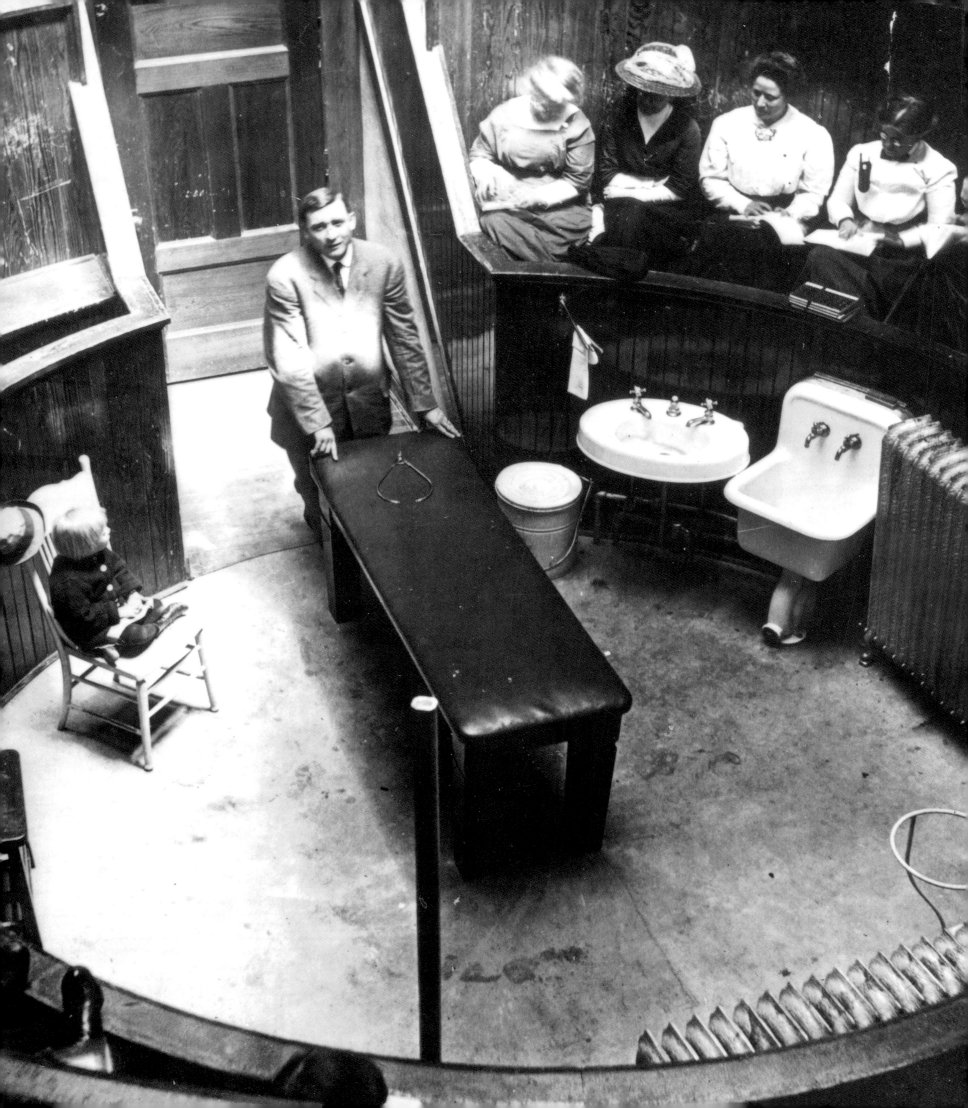

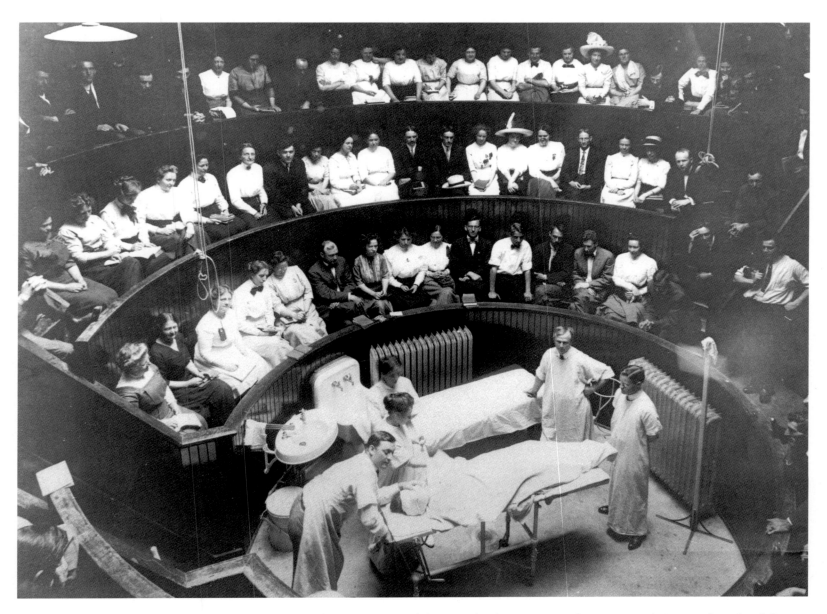

Left: *"The pit," an operating theater in the A. T. Still Surgical Sanitarium, provided a venue for the instructors to demonstrate techniques to the student body.*

Above: *Students observe a clinical demonstration in "the pit" with George Laughlin, DO (second from right), circa 1910.*

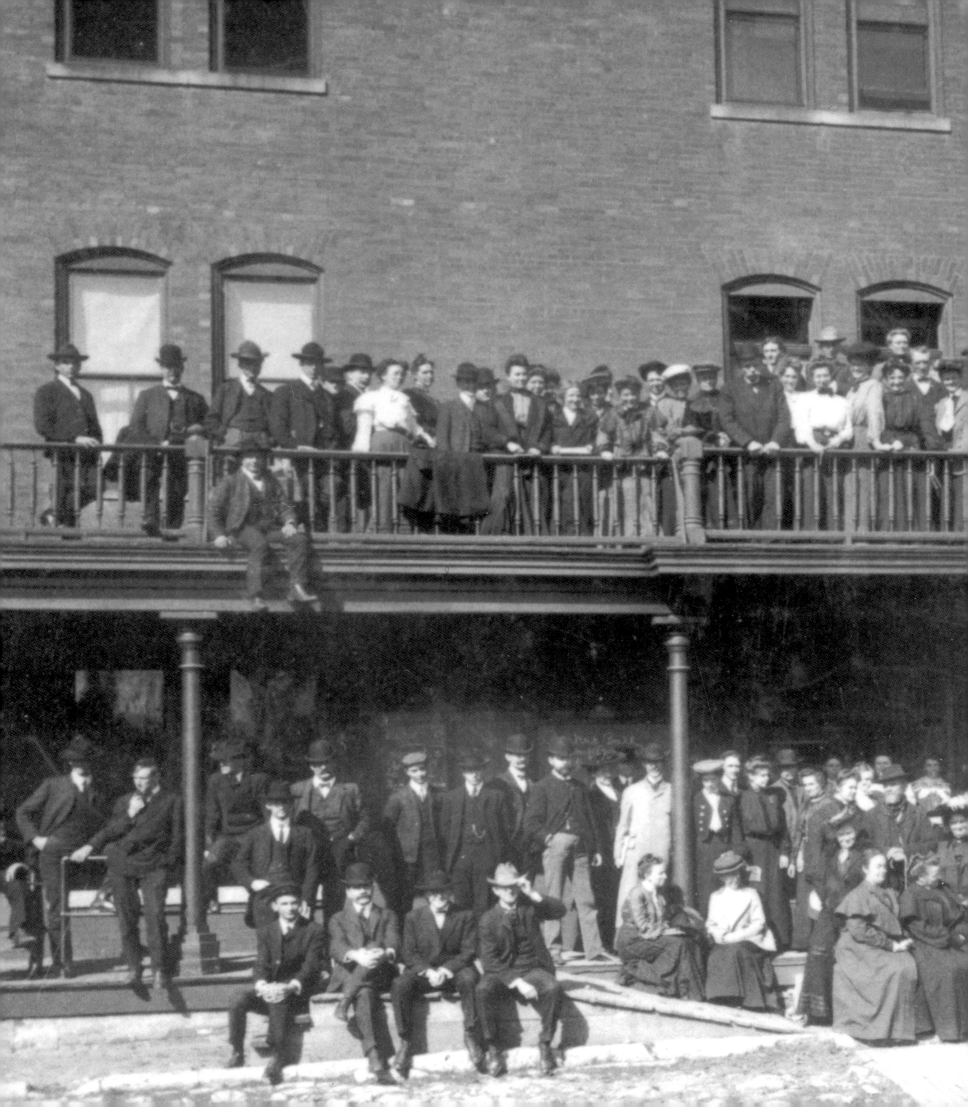

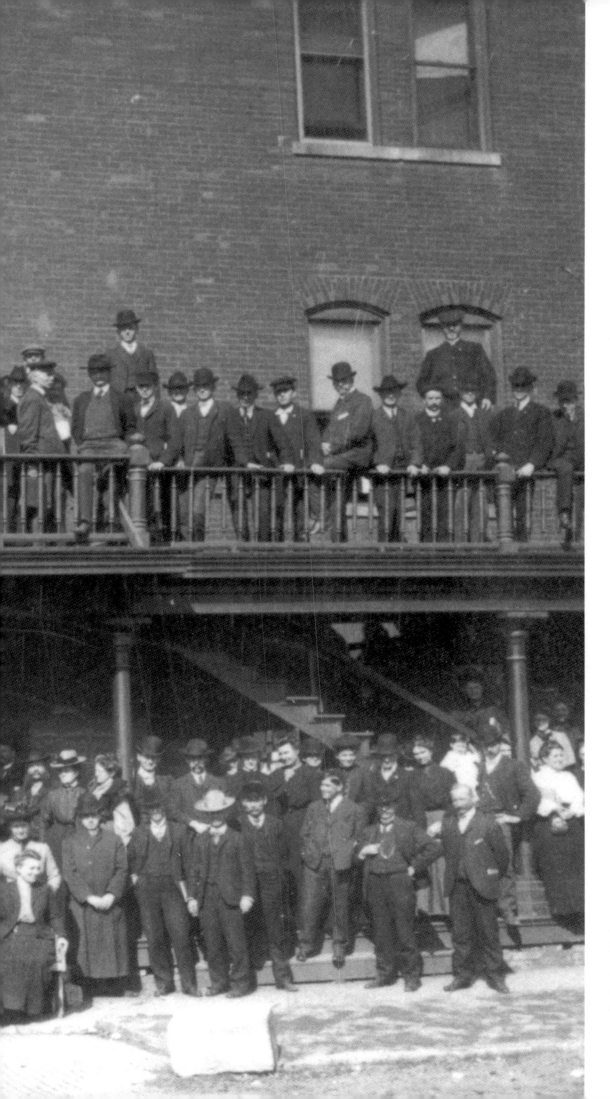

Left: The class of 1906, taken during its freshman year in 1904 in front of the A. T. Still Infirmary.

Overleaf: The American School of Osteopathy class of 1909 poses on the lawn of the Still mansion, with A. T. Still in the center, front.

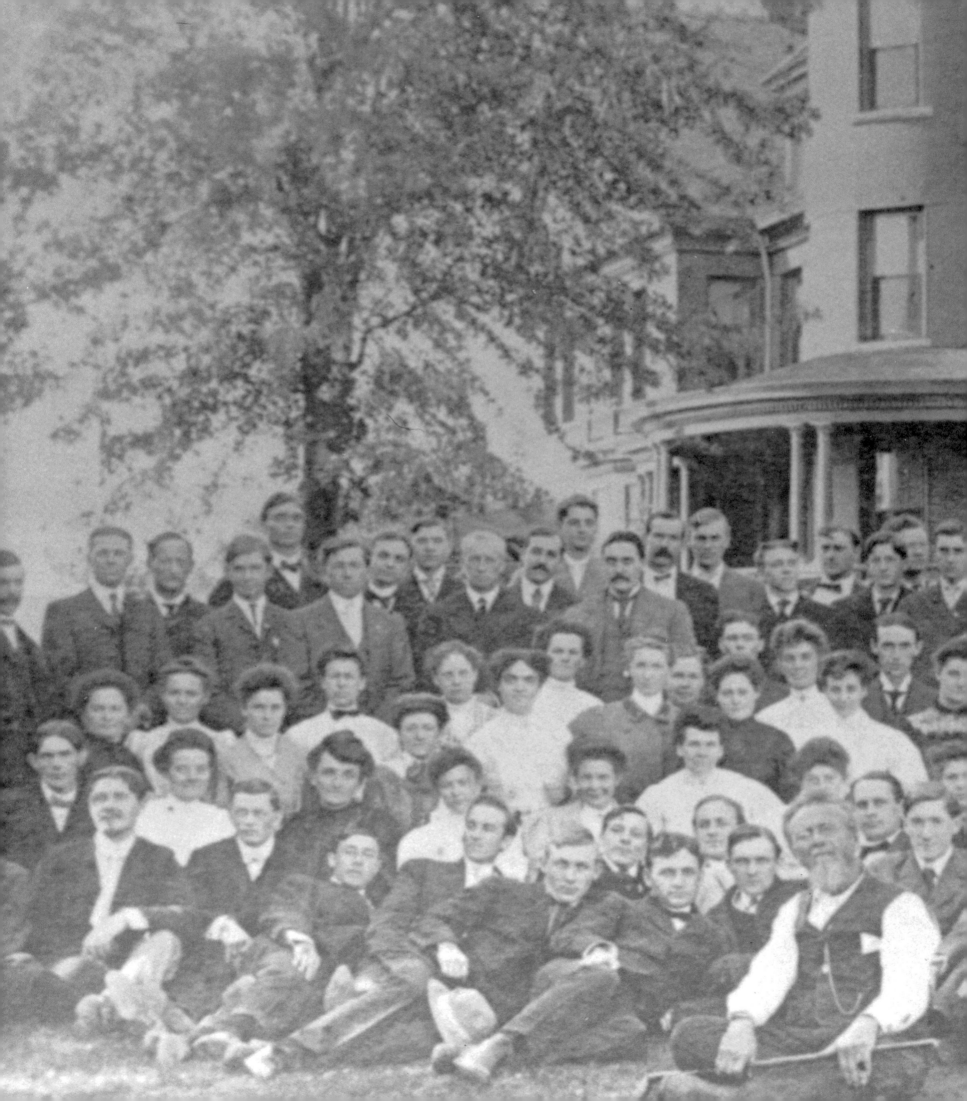

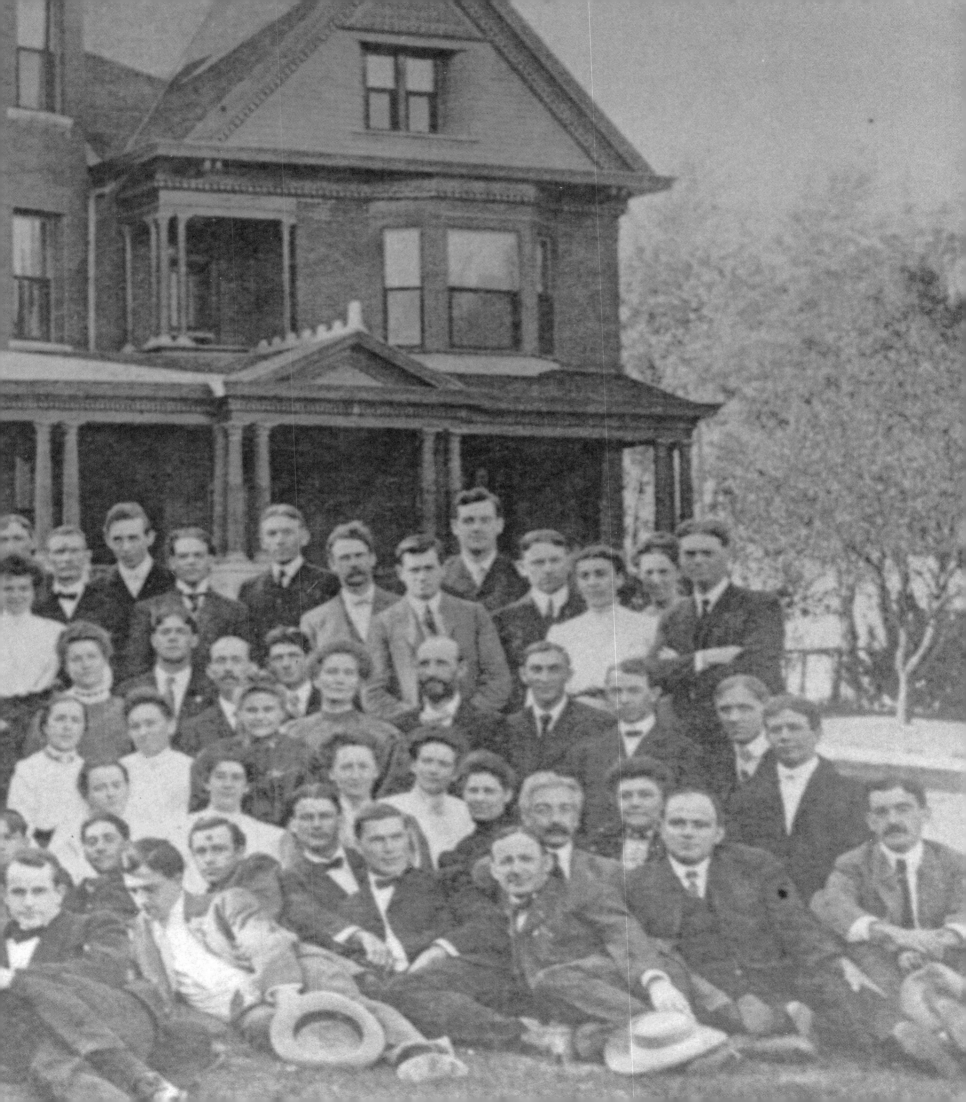

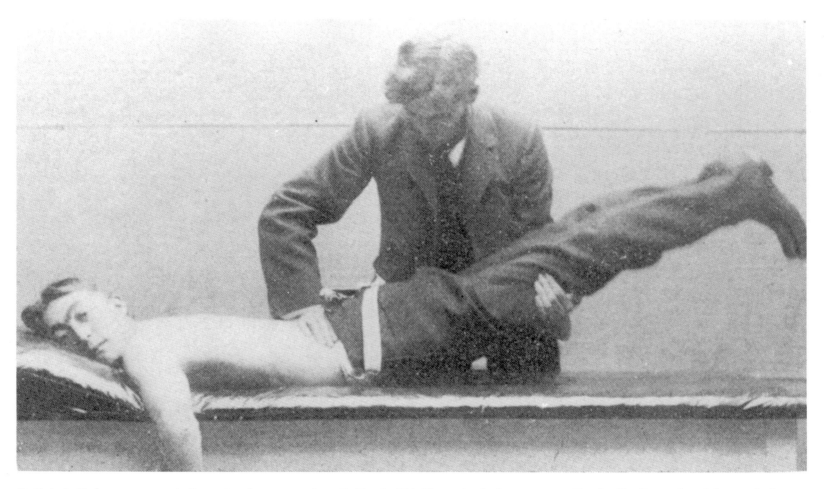

Dr Dain L. Tasker was among the first to introduce osteopathy to California. This illustration depicts treatment of lumbar disorders as described in Tasker's Principles of Osteopathy *(1902).*

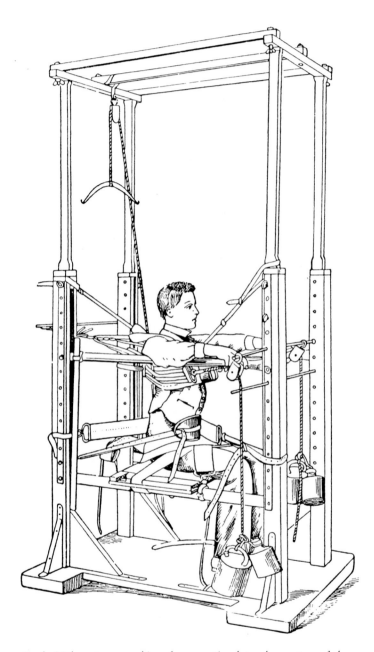

Early 20th-century machines for correcting lateral curvature of the spine looked very impressive but were not necessarily as effective.

A. T. Still was known as an agreeable photographic subject. He posed with each graduating class of the American School of Osteopathy and with the annual dissection classes until his death in 1917, and also enjoyed being the subject of less formal photographs.

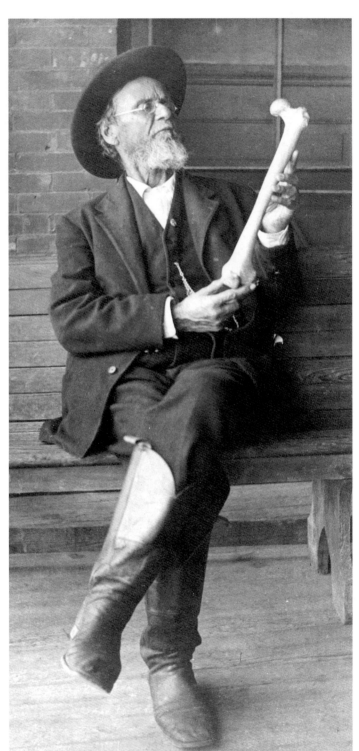

Right: *Dr Still was well known for carrying bone specimens such as this femur, which he used as subjects of study and demonstration.*

Far right: *Dr Still poses with Pearl Schreve and an unidentified woman, circa 1909.*

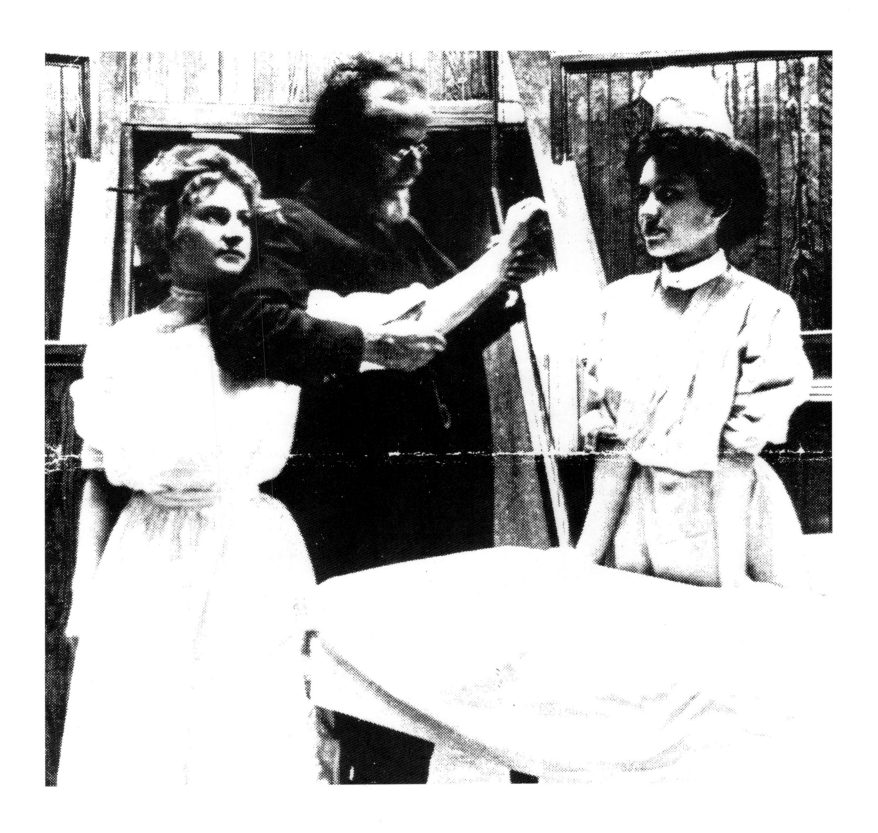

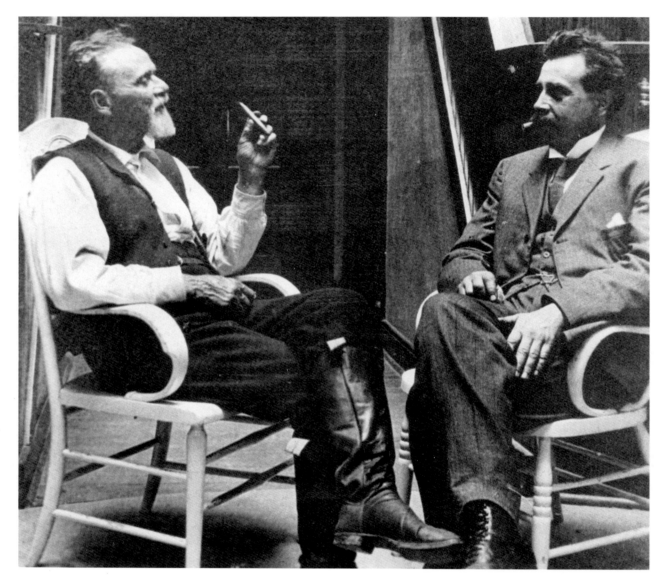

Dr Still and William Smith, MD, DO, pose in a relaxed manner in the surgical pit at the A. T. Still Surgical Sanitarium.

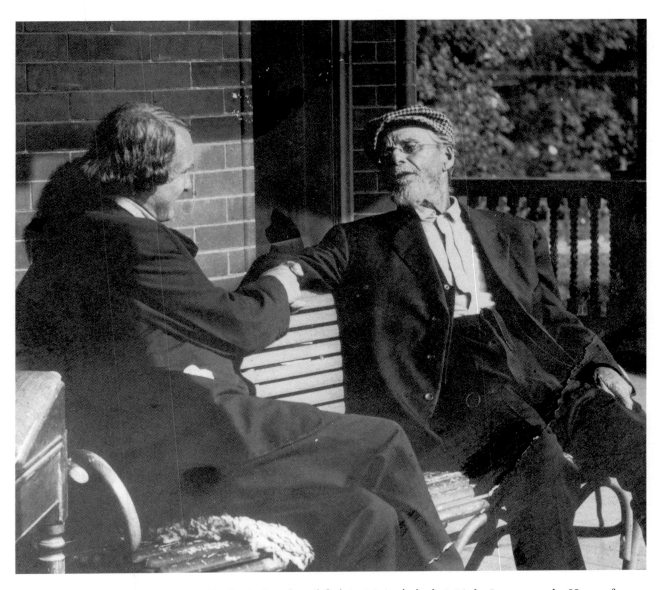

Dr Still relaxes with author Elbert Hubbard, who later described their visit in the book, A Little Journey to the Home of Andrew Taylor Still.

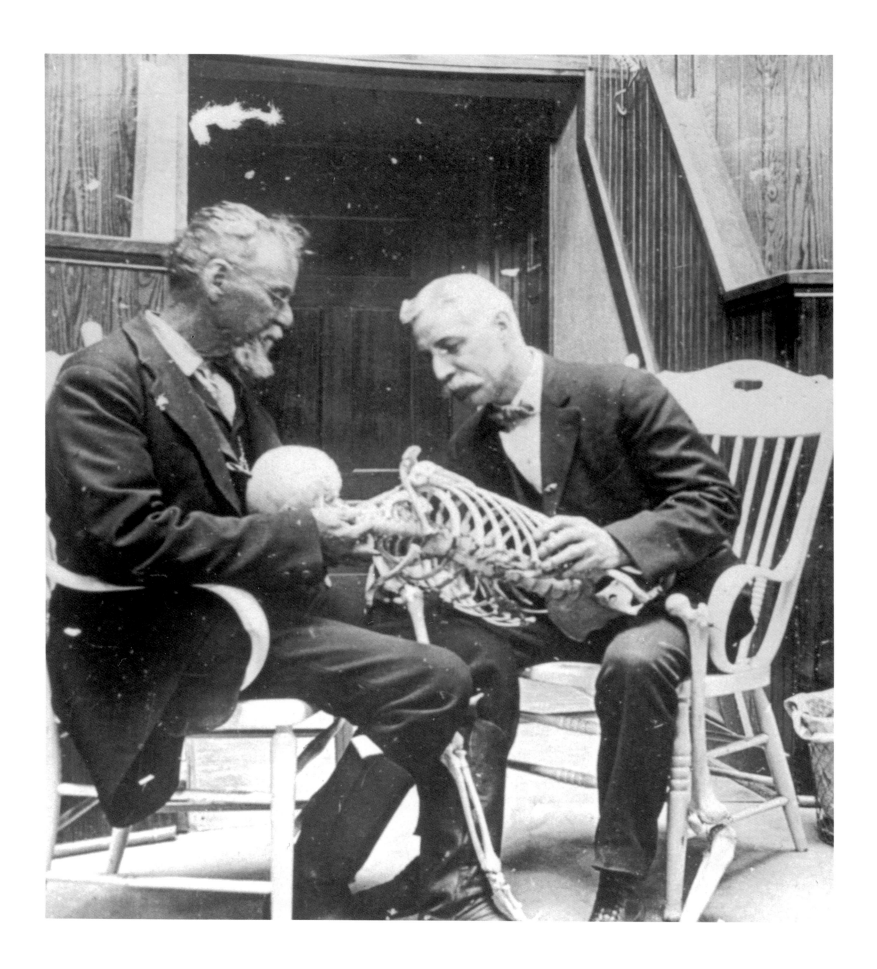

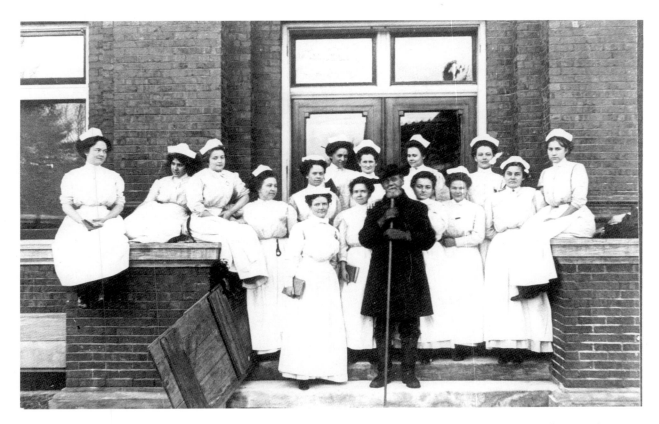

Left: *Dr Still and Dr FG Cluett, with demonstration skeleton, circa 1910, in the surgical pit at the A. T. Still Surgical Sanitarium.*

Above: *Nurses of the American School of Osteopathy hospital with A. T. Still on the hospital front steps, 1910-11.*

The period between 1910 and 1920 was marked by rapid growth and progress in osteopathic education and in the osteopathic profession. Osteopathic physicians organized more and more osteopathic organizations at the state and local levels, while the American Osteopathic Association flourished. Spurred on by the caustic 1910 report of Dr Abraham Flexner, osteopathy (and American allopathic medicine, too) evolved rapidly. Admissions criteria were tightened, and the instruction required for graduation increased during the decade until by 1916 the osteopathic curriculum consisted of a full 4-year course of study.

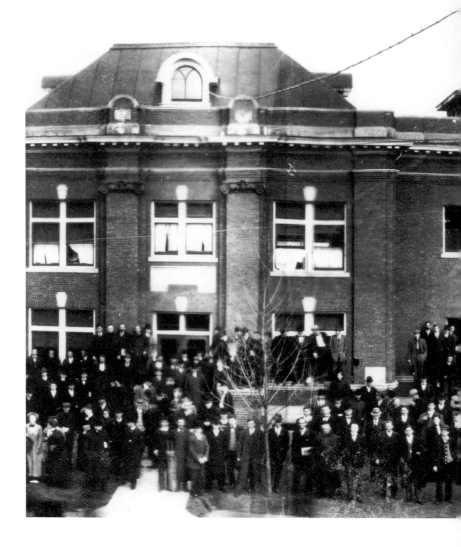

The American School of Osteopathy school and hospital around 1910.

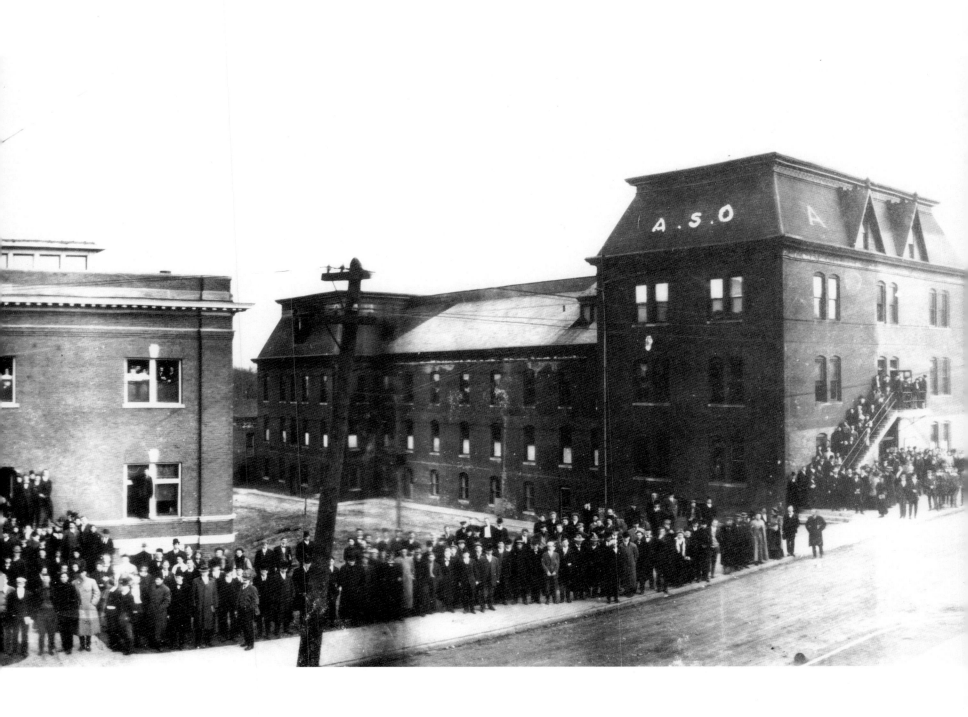

THE
WABASH ⬧ ROUTE

RUNS

4 Daily Passenger Trains into Kirksville! 4

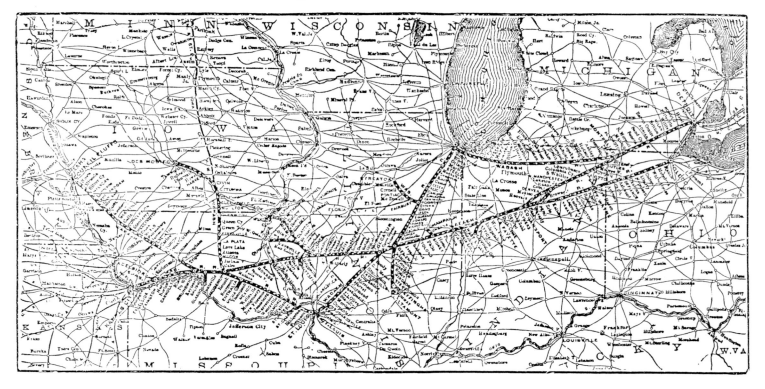

Making Close Connections with All Lines, and Giving
to the Public Excellent Service.

For the Benefit of Patients of the A. T. STILL INFIRMARY,
this Road Has Placed on Sale

Special Rate Tickets at One Fare for the Round Trip

from all Points Between Moberly, Mo., and Ottumwa, Iowa.

Address   **W. E. NOONAN,** Agent, Kirksville, Mo.

C. S. CRANE, General Passenger and Ticket Agent, St. Louis, Mo.

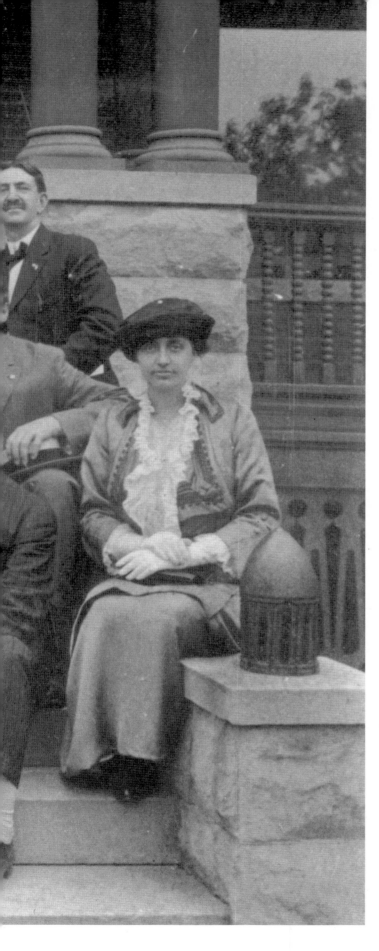

In 1915, past presidents of the American Osteopathic Association posed on the steps of the Still mansion, with Dr Still seated in the center, rear.

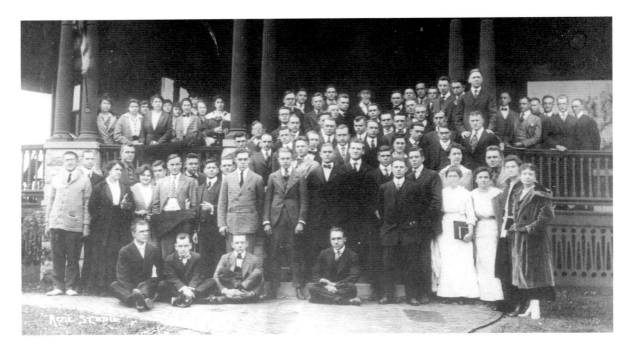

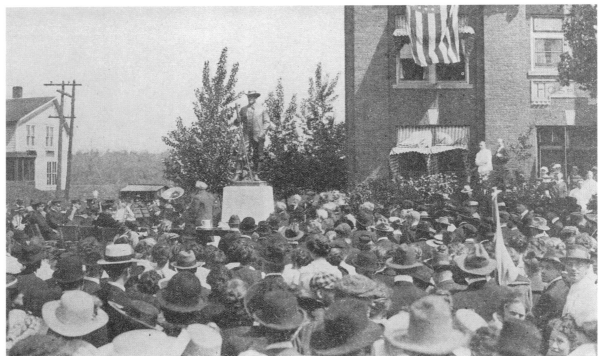

Above: The 1917 graduating class of the American School of Osteopathy was the last class to pose with Dr Still, seen in the center, rear.

Below: Charles Still, Jr, presided over the unveiling of the George Zolnay statue of his grandfather, A. T. Still, on May 23, 1917, shortly before the elder Still's death.

Right: The Zolnay statue of A. T. Still now stands at the Adair County Courthouse in Kirksville, Missouri.

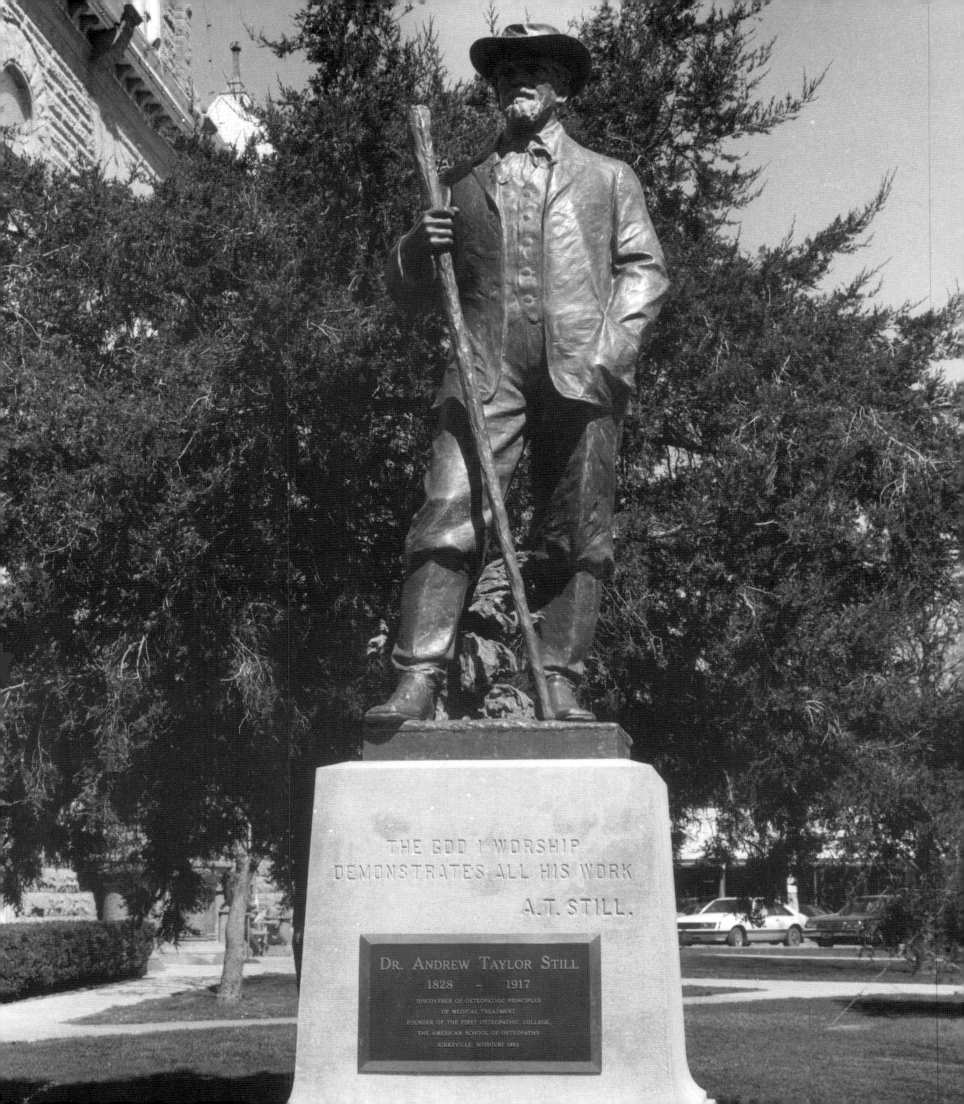

THE GOD I WORSHIP
DEMONSTRATES ALL HIS WORK
A.T. STILL.

DR. ANDREW TAYLOR STILL
1828 – 1917
DISCOVERER OF OSTEOPATHIC PRINCIPLES
OF MEDICAL TREATMENT
FOUNDER OF THE FIRST OSTEOPATHIC COLLEGE,
THE AMERICAN SCHOOL OF OSTEOPATHY
KIRKSVILLE, MISSOURI 1892

In 1918 there occurred a worldwide epidemic of type B influenza. Mortality from the influenza and complications such as pneumonia were very high. Osteopathic medicine rose to the occasion and delivered care to the suffering. Leading the way, staff from the ASO worked with the Red Cross in Kirksville to establish an ad hoc Influenza Hospital. Reported results from osteopaths around the country suggested that osteopathic treatment of these diseases produced results favorable in every way compared to those from allopathic treatment. Many of the experiences of osteopathic physicians during the 1918 influenza pandemic are recounted in a series of letters compiled and published as "Experiences With the Epidemic" in the *Journal of the American Osteopathic Association.*

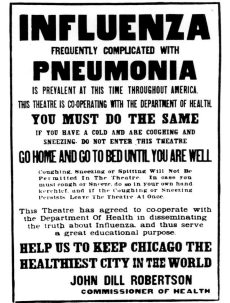

INFLUENZA
FREQUENTLY COMPLICATED WITH
PNEUMONIA
IS PREVALENT AT THIS TIME THROUGHOUT AMERICA.
THIS THEATRE IS CO-OPERATING WITH THE DEPARTMENT OF HEALTH.
YOU MUST DO THE SAME
IF YOU HAVE A COLD AND ARE COUGHING AND
SNEEZING. DO NOT ENTER THIS THEATRE
GO HOME AND GO TO BED UNTIL YOU ARE WELL
Coughing, Sneezing or Spitting Will Not Be
Permitted In The Theatre. In case you
must cough or Sneeze, do so in your own hand
kerchief, and if the Coughing or Sneezing
Persists Leave The Theatre At Once.

This Theatre has agreed to co-operate with
the Department Of Health in disseminating
the truth about Influenza, and thus serve
a great educational purpose.

**HELP US TO KEEP CHICAGO THE
HEALTHIEST CITY IN THE WORLD**
JOHN DILL ROBERTSON
COMMISSIONER OF HEALTH

Left: Public health departments across the country issued advisories in an attempt to prevent the spread of influenza.

Right: The growing osteopathic profession also received recognition and support from influential persons such as Theodore Roosevelt, Samuel Clemens, and Eddie Rickenbacker.

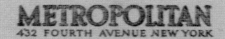

METROPOLITAN
432 FOURTH AVENUE NEW YORK

Office of
Theodore Roosevelt

December 13, 1917.

My dear Dr. Green:

I wish the American Osteopathic
Association all success in its effort to secure for
osteopathic physicians the right to serve their country
in the army and navy.   I am sorry that licensed osteopathic physicians who have passed the Medical Examining
Board examinations for commissions on the Medical Corps
and have been recommended by the Examining Board for such
commissions have not received them.   I am glad that the
American Osteopathic Association is patriotically endeavor-
ing without cost to the men, to give them osteopathic care
in the camps and cantonments.   I earnestly hope that
Congress will pass legislation enabling Osteopathic Physicians
to serve their country in the capacity for which they are
best fitted.

I write on this subject with knowledge.
Two of the members of my family have been treated with
great profit to themselves for years by Osteophatic Physicians.
One of these is now with our army in France. It would be to
his great advantage if he could have occasional osteopathic
treatments, and I am genuinely concerned that he is unable
to get them.   To give Osteophatic Physicians the chance to
serve the army in the country as you desire would be a
very real benefit.

With all good wishes,

Faithfully yours,

Theodore Roosevelt -
You are welcome to use this
in any way you wish.

The 1920s was a decade of growth for the American Osteopathic Association. The nation prospered, and so did osteopathic physicians. The scope of activities of the association increased, its staff grew and developed, and the organization enjoyed financial success. Membership increased, and publications such as the *Journal of the AOA*, *Osteopathic Health*, and *Osteopathic Forum* became a major source of revenue. The annual conventions increased in size and popularity.

Following the stock market crash of 1929, a decade of difficulty began for osteopathic physicians, and the economic plight of the nation spelled trouble for the American Osteopathic Association. Yet skillful management saved the organization from ruin, and it moved through the Great Depression and into a brighter future.

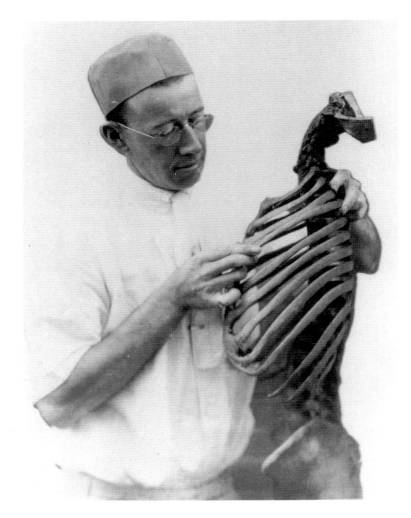

Right: A. Virgil "Spine" Halladay, DO, demonstrates his famous Halladay Flexible Spine. Dr Halladay developed a process in which the spine was removed from a cadaver and treated with preservative chemicals in such a manner that it retained lifelike flexibility. This proved a very useful teaching aid in anatomic instruction.

Far right: Two students dissected and mounted this complete human nervous system in 1925 at the American School of Osteopathy, a task that required more than 100 hours of dissection. M. A. Schlack and L. P. Ransdell not only passed anatomy, but later served as faculty at that school. The specimen is on permanent exhibit at the Still National Osteopathic Museum.

Overleaves: The 1928 American Osteopathic Association convention, held at Kirksville, Missouri, commemorated the centennial of A. T. Still's birth. This major celebration attracted osteopathic physicians from across the country.

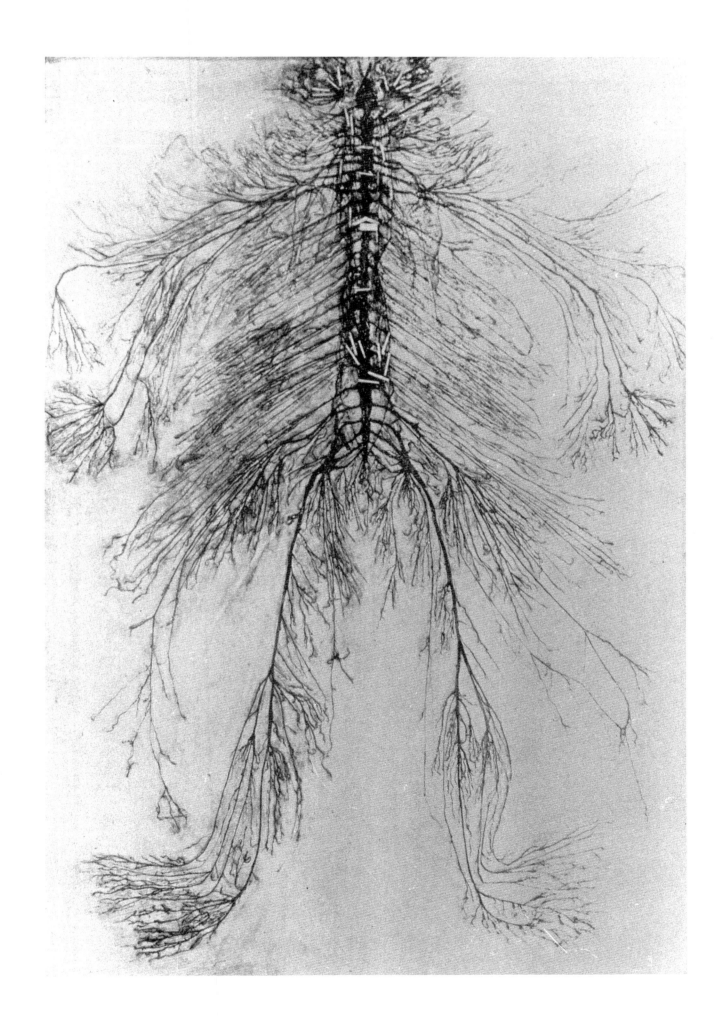

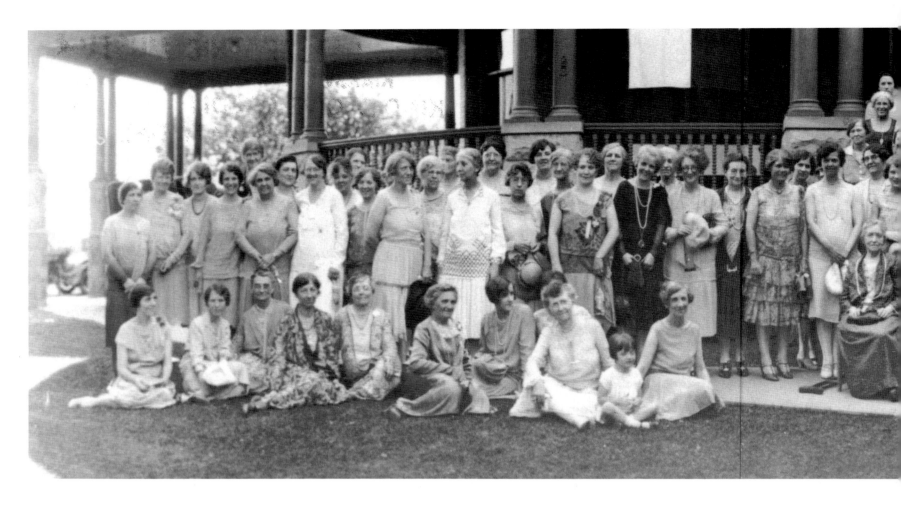

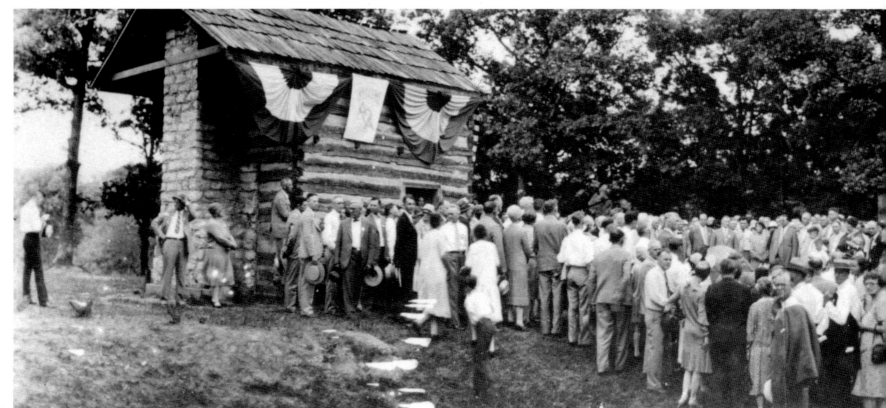

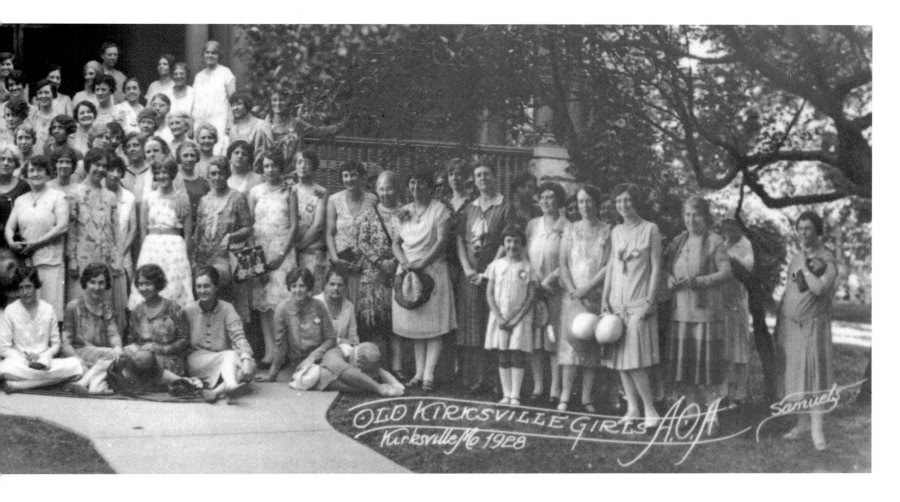

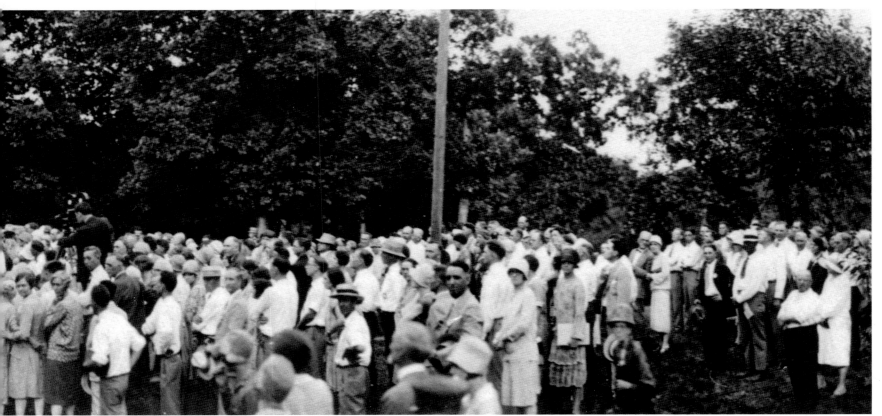

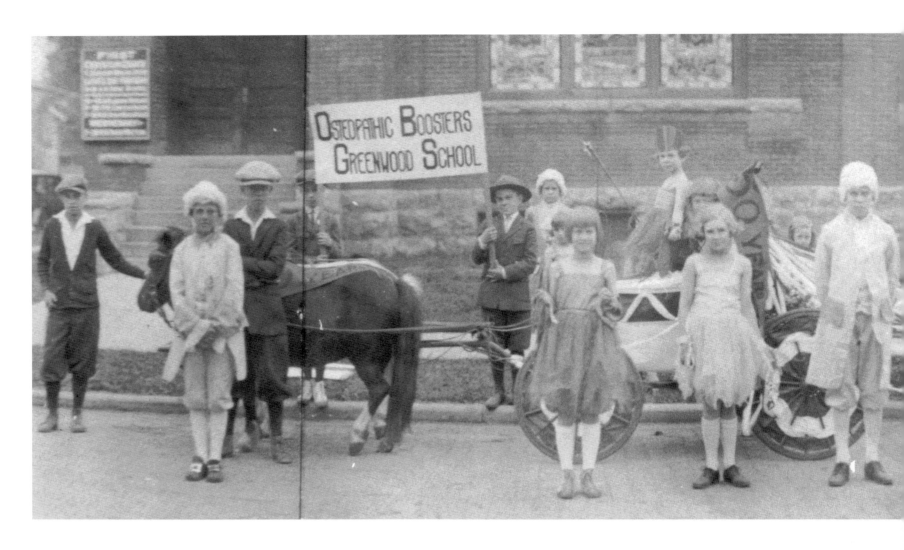

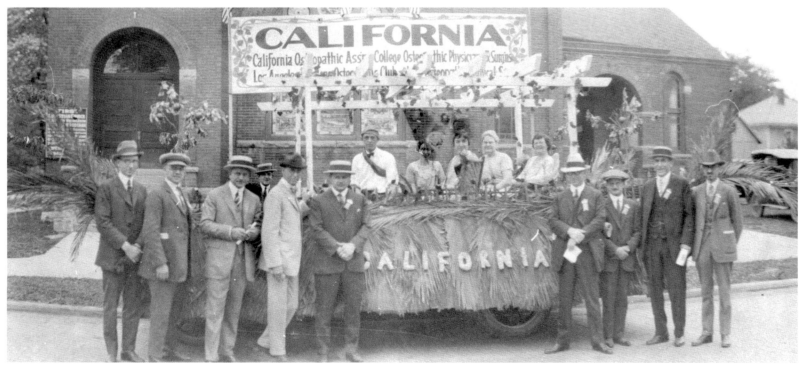

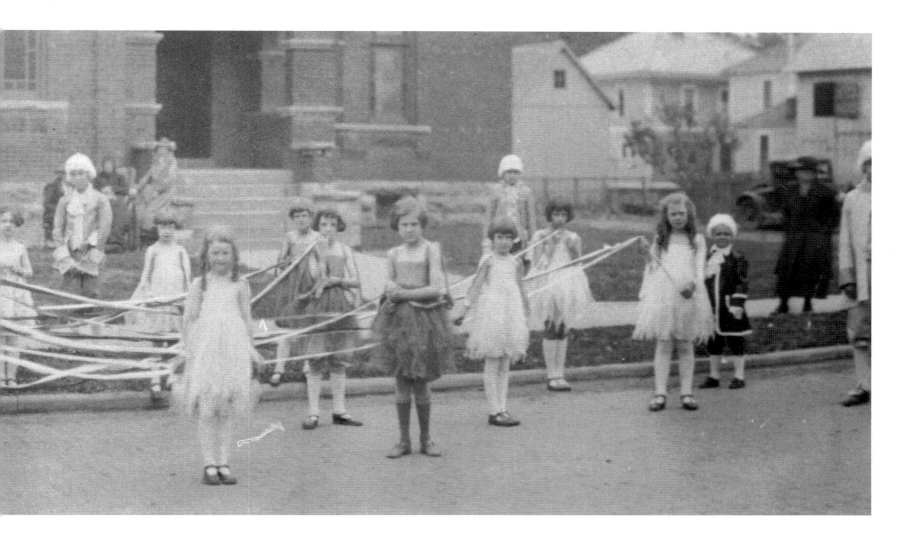

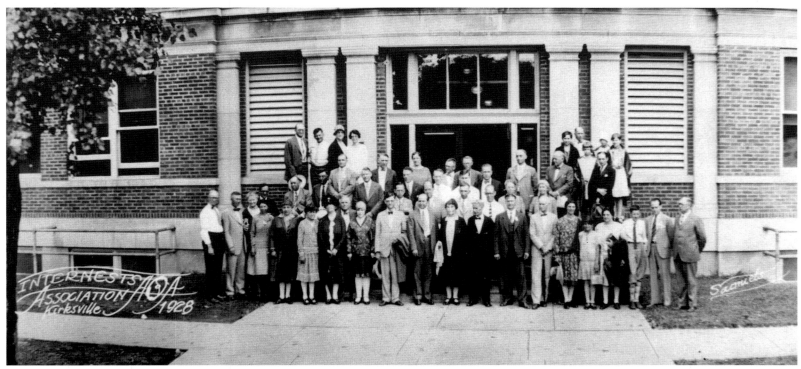

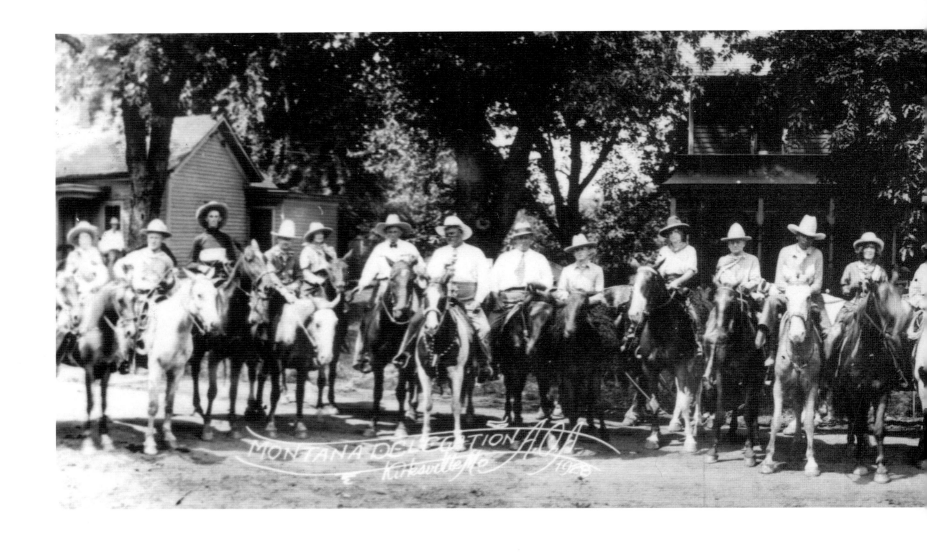

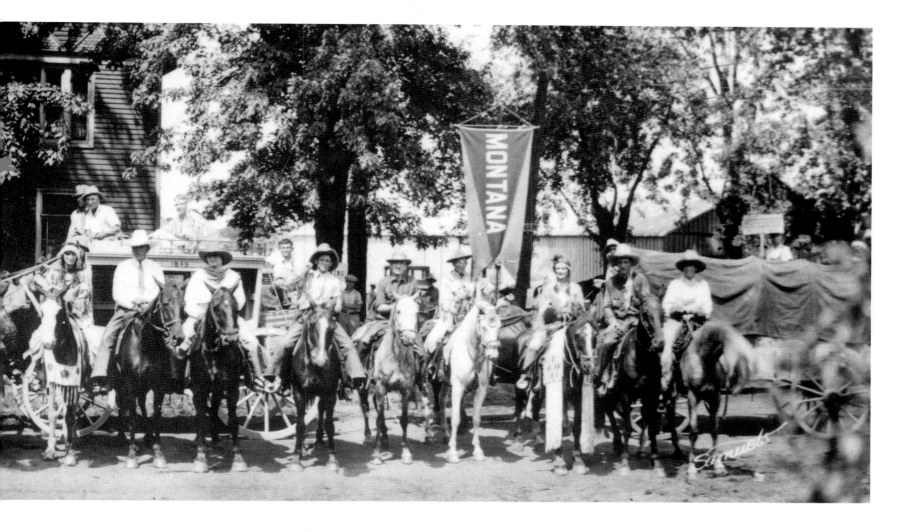

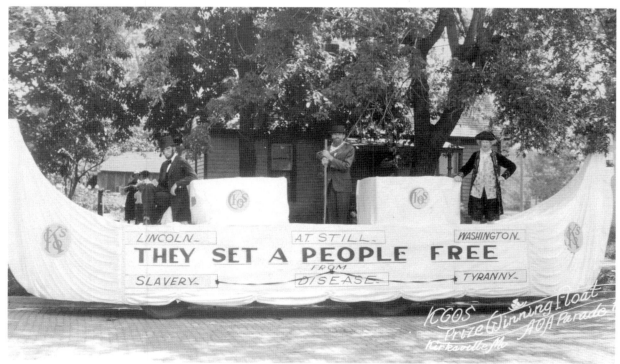

LINCOLN. A.T. STILL. WASHINGTON.
THEY SET A PEOPLE FREE
FROM
SLAVERY. DISEASE. TYRANNY.

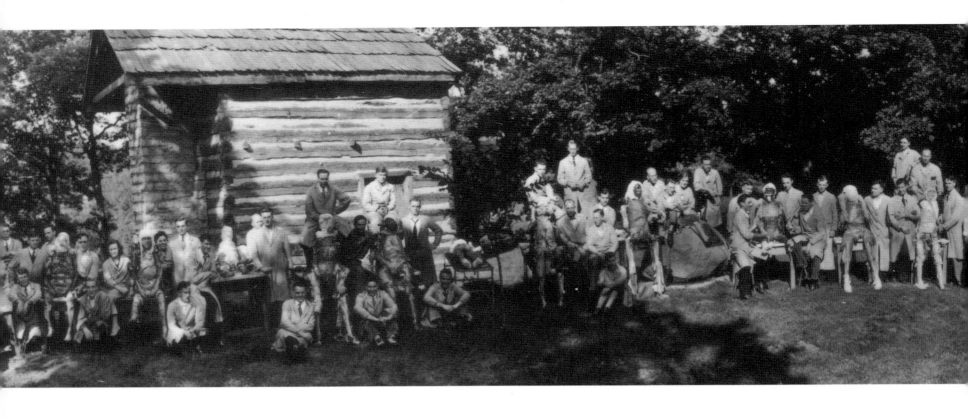

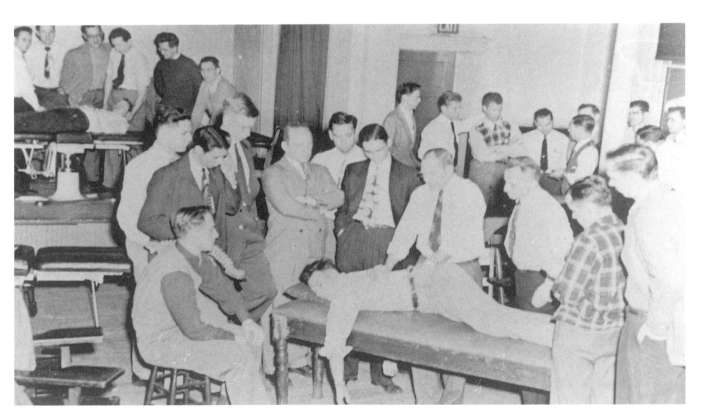

D. A class in osteopathic manipulation at the Chicago College of Osteopathic Medicine, 1957.

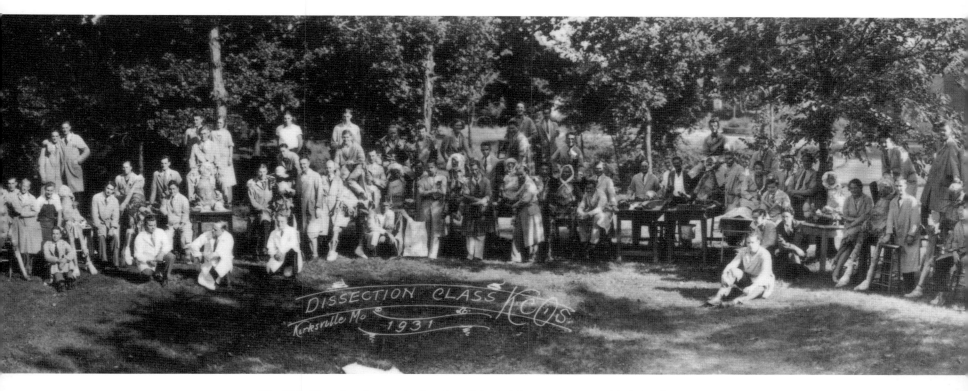

The 1931 dissection class at the American School of Osteopathy poses with their cadavers.

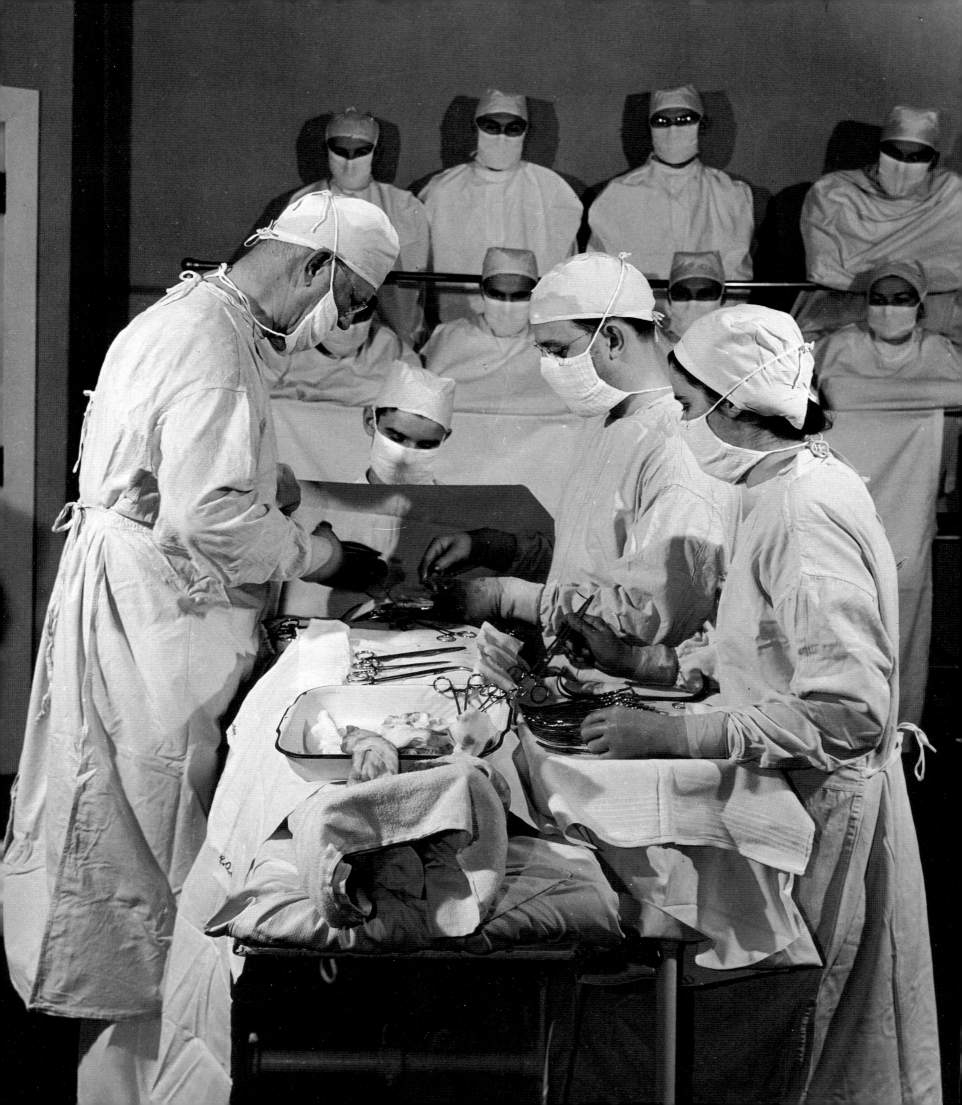

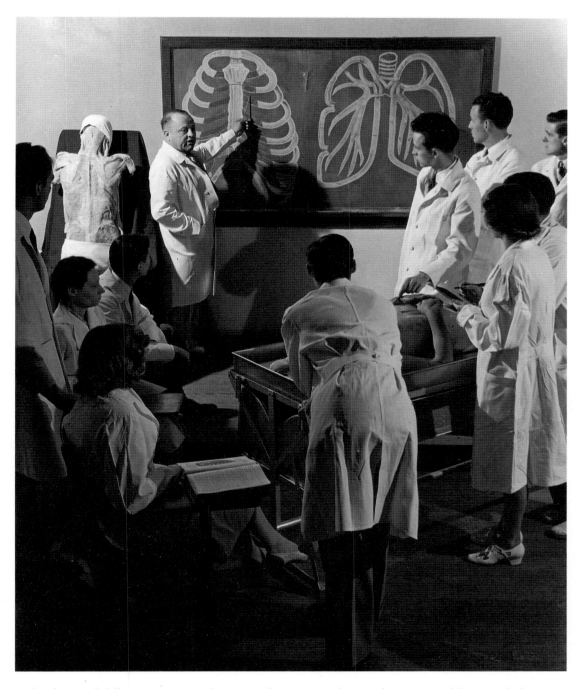

Left, above and following pages: *In the 1940s* Life *magazine photographer Otto Hagel documented the training of osteopathic physicians at the Kirksville College of Osteopathic Medicine.*

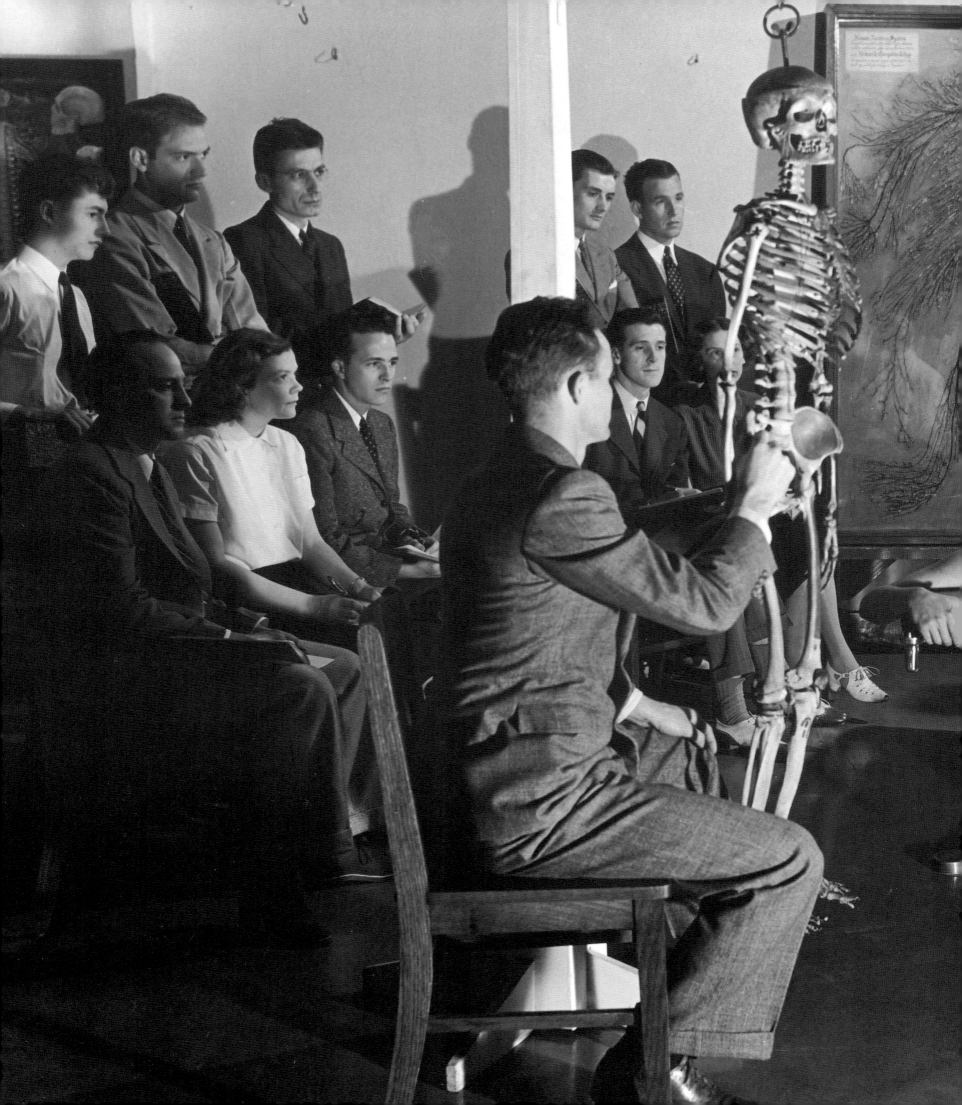

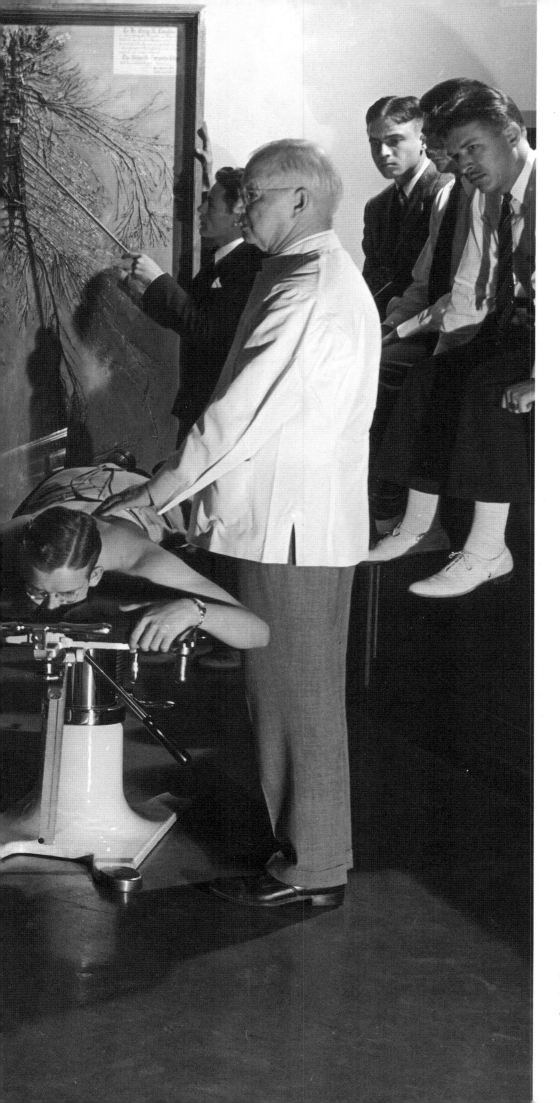

Overleaf: The forty-fifth annual convention of the American Osteopathic Association was held in Atlantic City, New Jersey, in 1941.

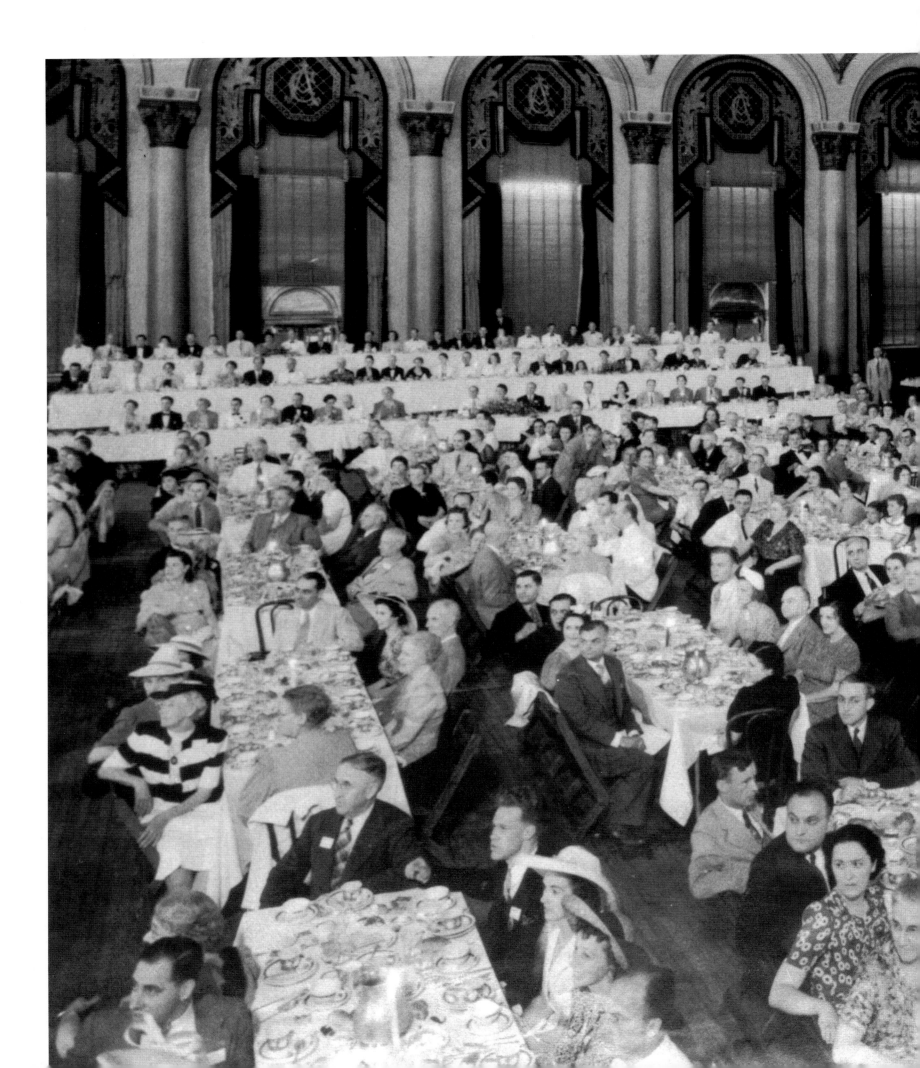

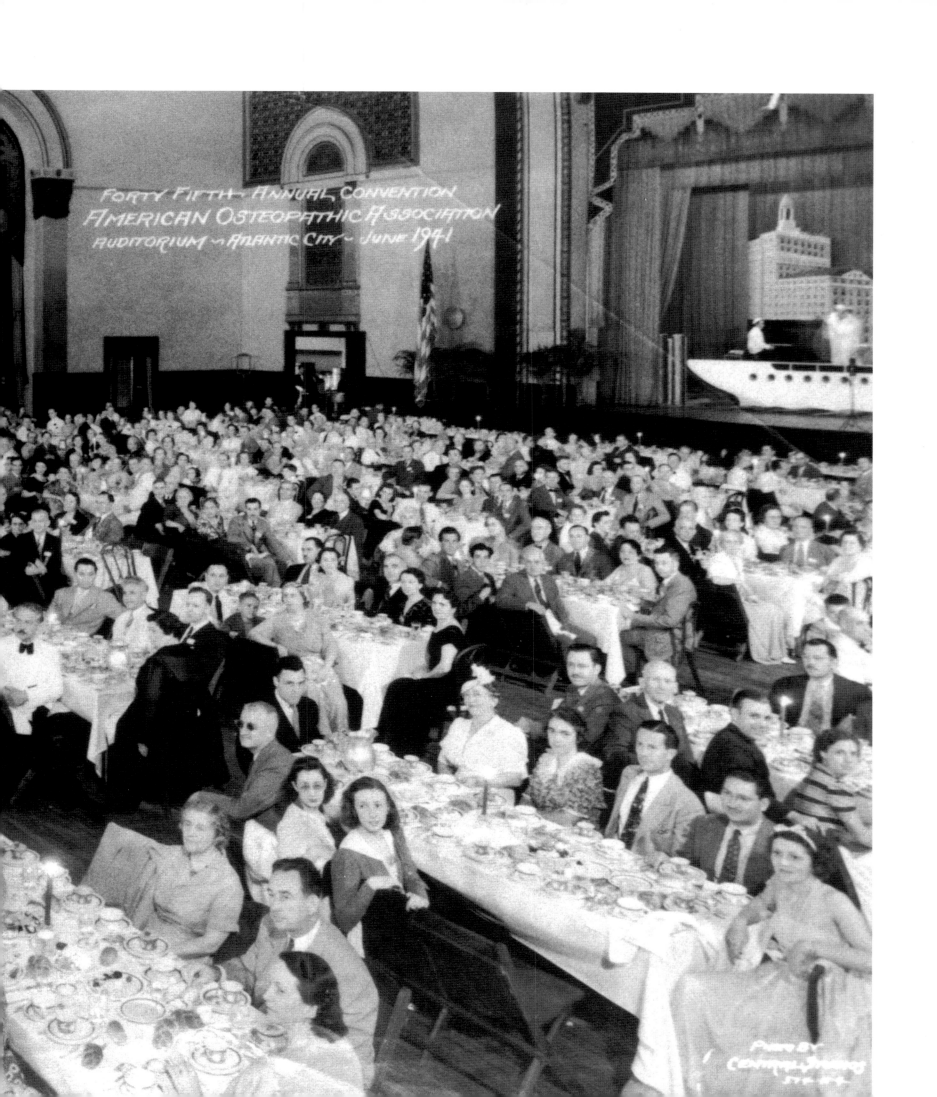

clinical Practice

Osteopathy began serving rural patients over a century ago, when Dr Still dedicated his practice to serving poor, working people. As an itinerant physician, he shared the science of osteopathy with the common men and women of his day. As his practice expanded, and house calls became a less effective use of his time, Dr Still established an office in downtown Kirksville. His practice there set a precedent that would later be followed by many other osteopathic physicians who made the small town clinic an osteopathic tradition.

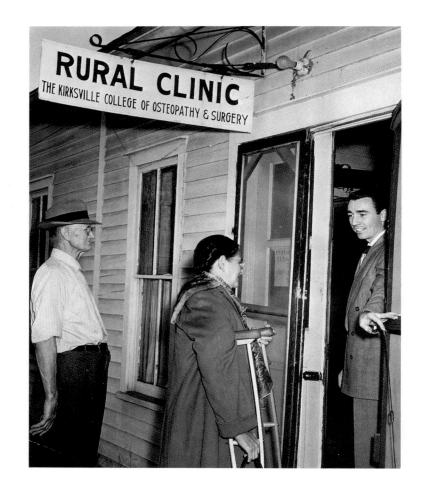

Right: *The Kirksville College opened its Rural Clinic Program in 1949. This innovative program provided rural access to quality osteopathic services, along with an opportunity for students to train in the community.*

Far right: *In the 1950s, clinic programs such as this one at Kirksville provided preschool physical examinations for local children.*

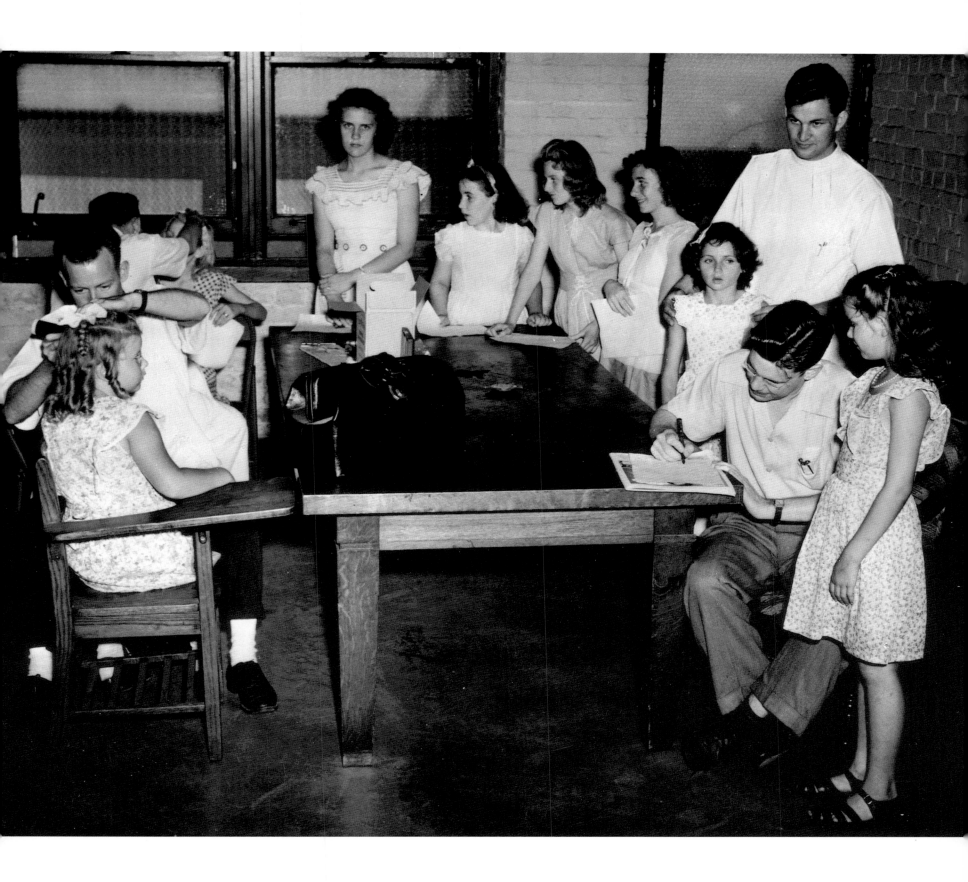

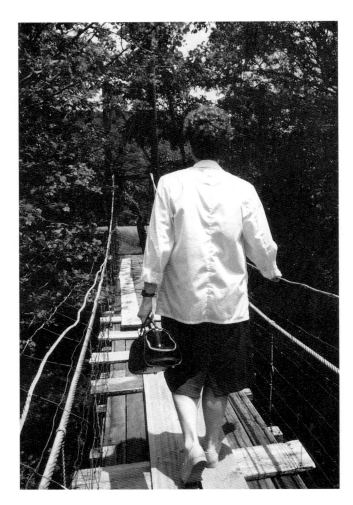

Above: Susan Debremaecker, DO, walks to the home of one of her patients in rural Althens, West Virginia. While DOs comprise 5% of US physicians, they make up 15% of doctors who serve rural areas and smaller communities.

Right: In the early 1980s, shortly after the New England school was founded, faculty and students traveled across Maine in the school's mobile medical unit, providing health screenings to rural, medically underserved areas.

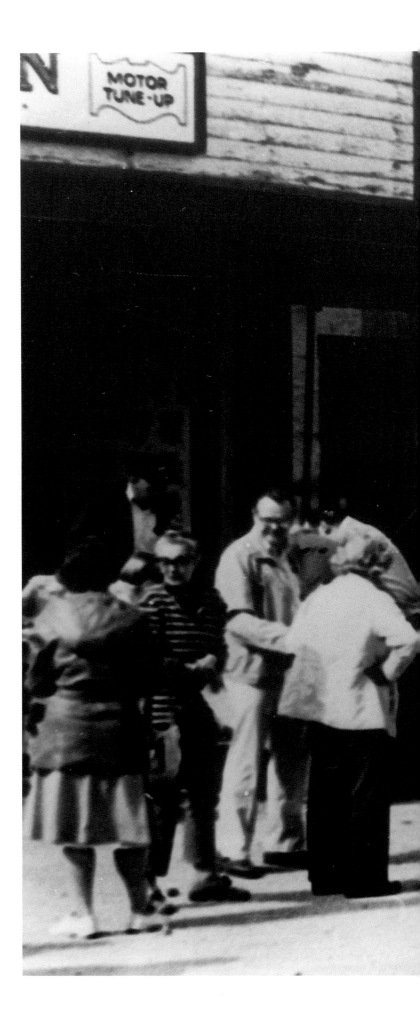

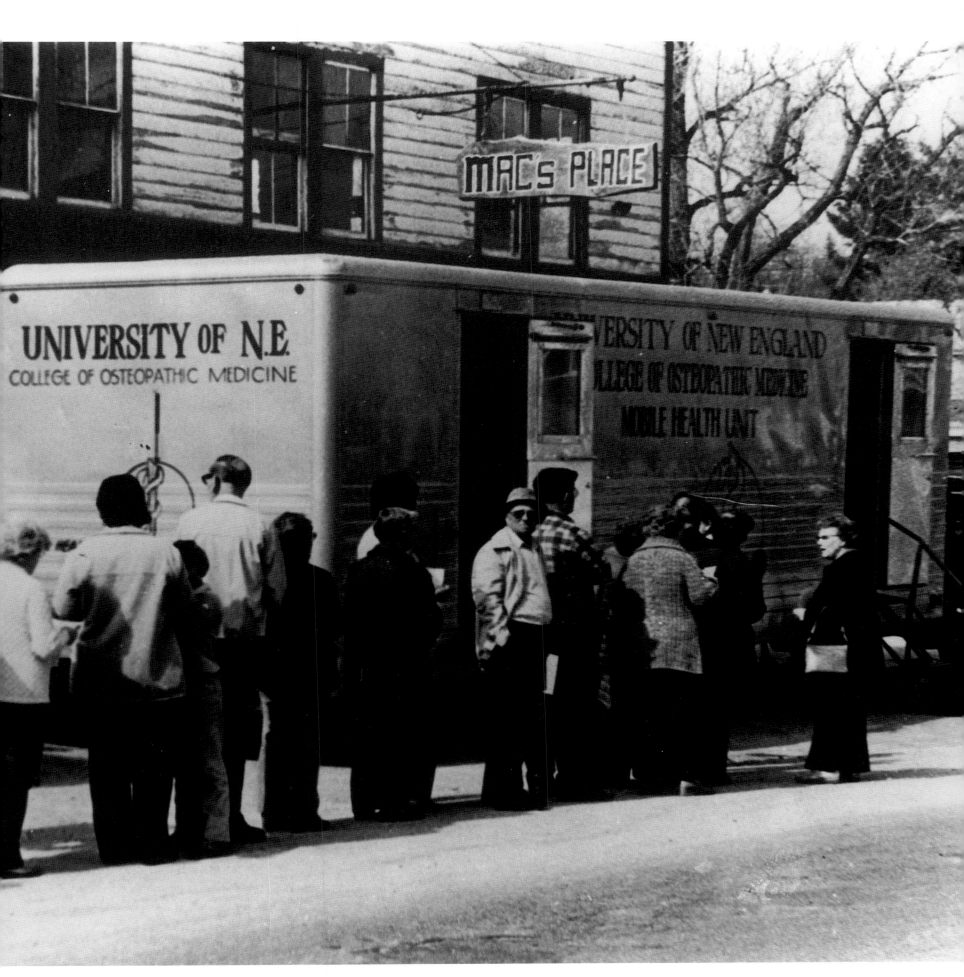

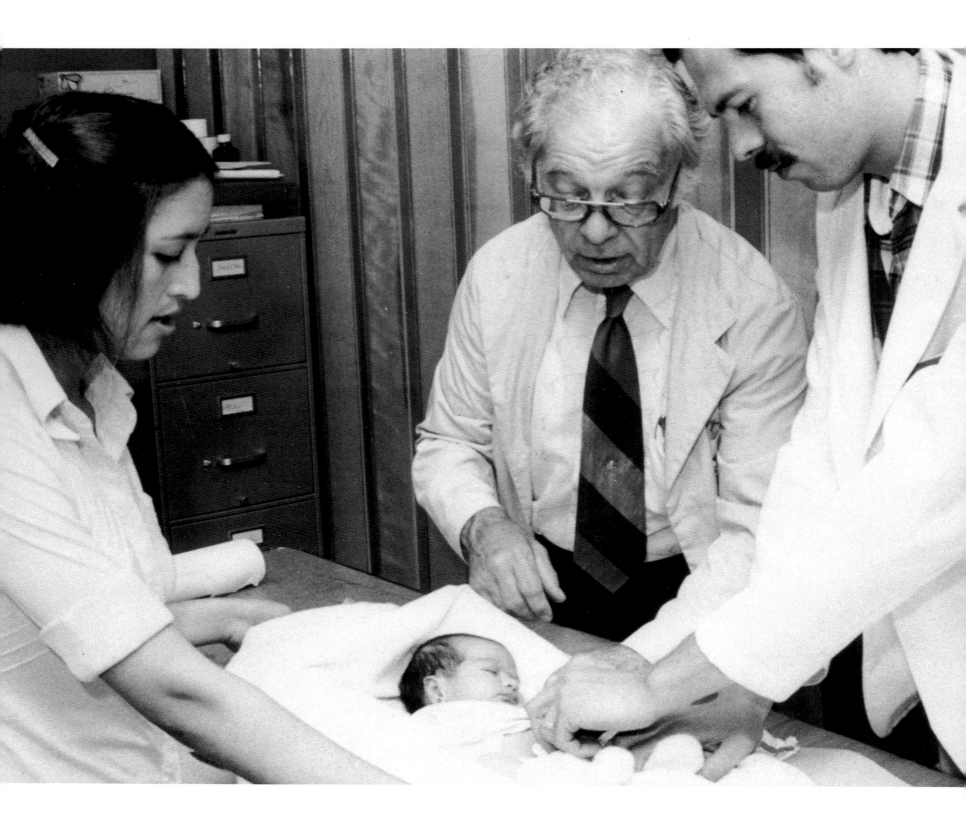

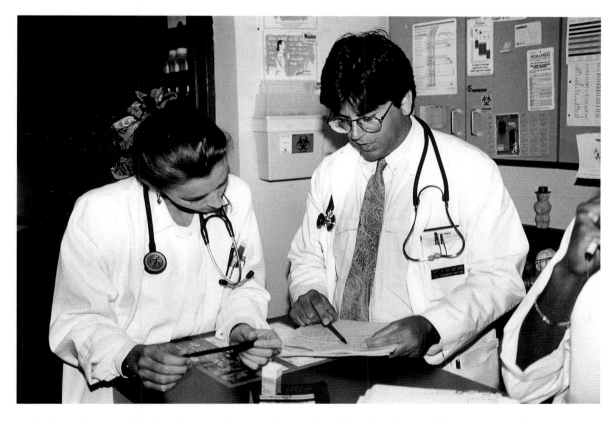

Left: In Michigan, a clinic for migrant workers provides much-needed medical care to this very poor population.

Above: The clinic is a mainstay for both practice and education in osteopathic medicine; it serves the community and, for the student, the clinic provides the experience of clinical rotation.

Although Dr Still remained in Kirksville, many of his students set up their own practices in urban areas. This allowed the development of osteopathic hospitals, in which osteopathic physicians of all specialties could practice.

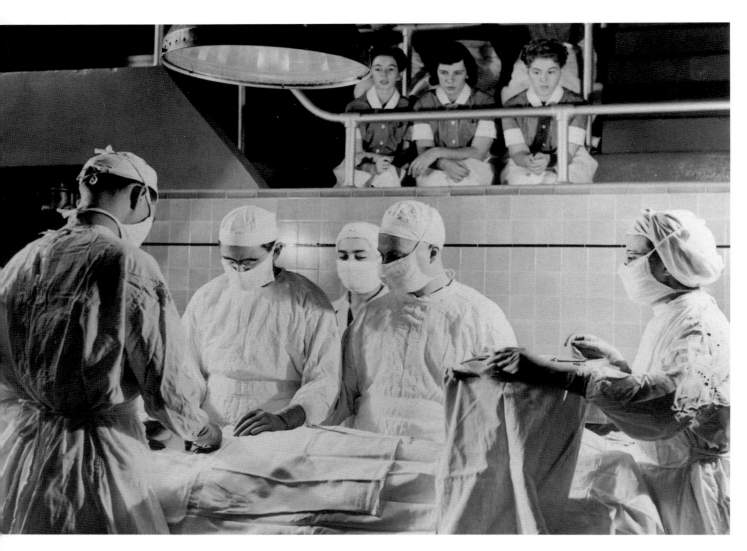

Above and right: One hundred forty osteopathic hospitals are accredited in the US. These institutions offer a wide variety of specialized medical services, including sophisticated surgical care.

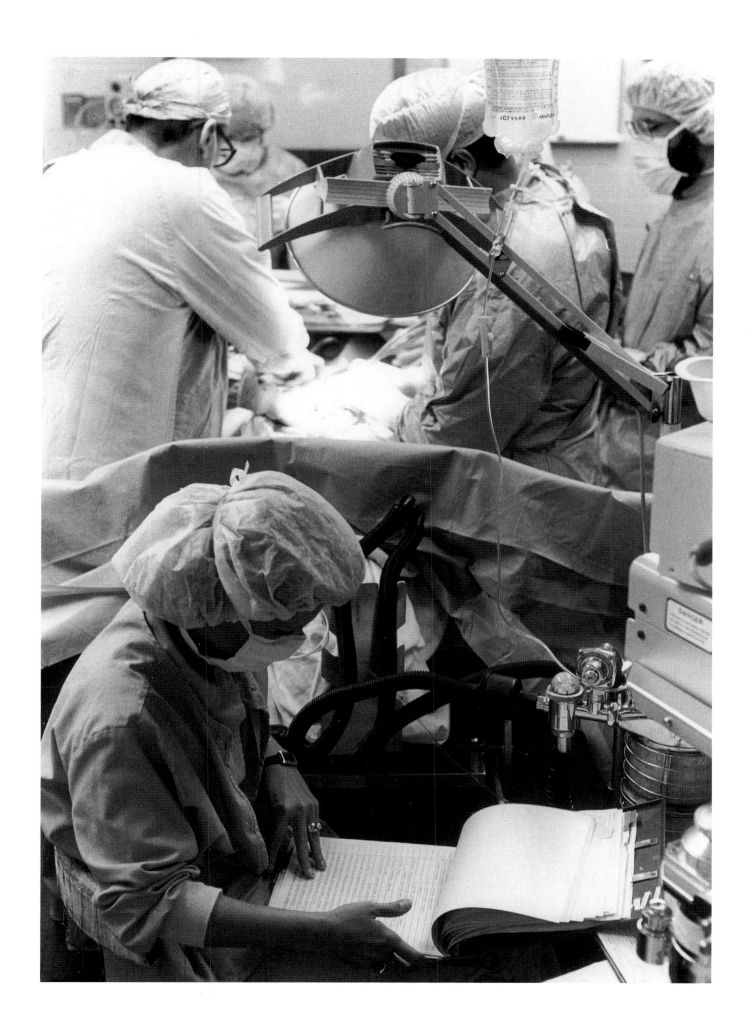

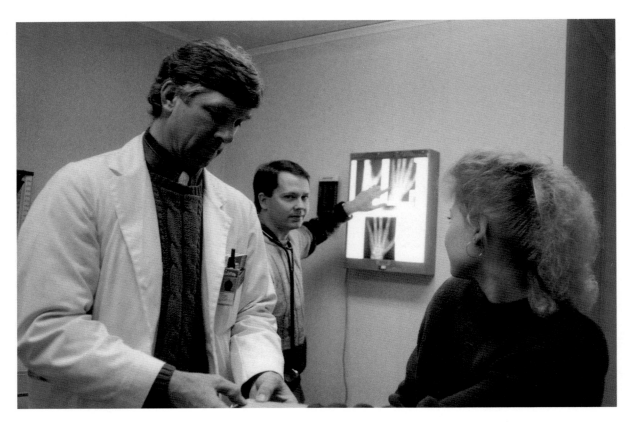

Just two years after Wilhelm Röntgen demonstrated his discovery of X-rays, the American School of Osteopathy purchased the largest model of X-ray machine available. X-rays continue to assist osteopathic physicians in making an accurate diagnosis.

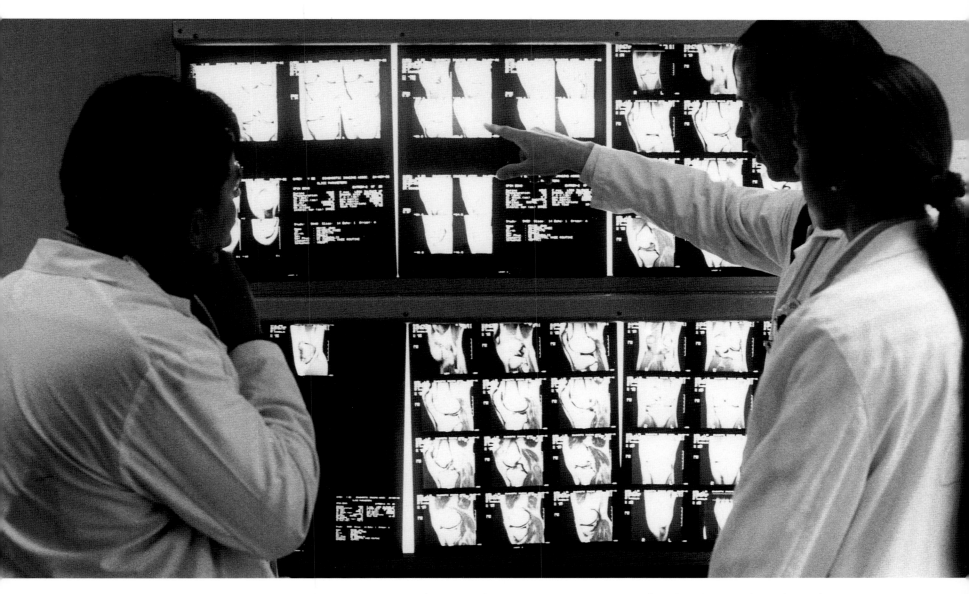

As diagnostic imaging increases in sophistication, so its value increases in osteopathic diagnosis. Here at the New York College of Osteopathic Medicine physicians use magnetic resonance imaging to diagnose many disorders.

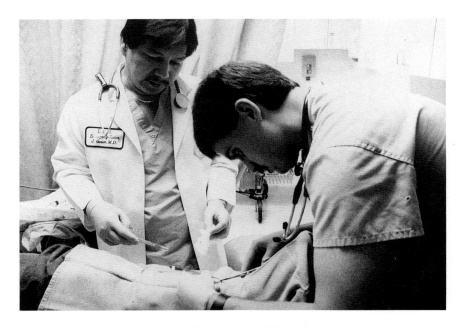

Above: *Emergency rooms, such as this one in rural West Virginia, present many opportunities for allopathic and osteopathic physicians to work side by side.*

Right: *Although Dr Still was opposed to using the addictive medication available a century ago, the tradition of osteopathic treatment has long included the administration of prescription medications. Shown are M. Chet Suske, DO, President of the Maine Osteopathic Association; Tom Nichols, District Sales Manager, Allen & Hanburys; and Fred Montgomery, Executive Sales Representative, Allen & Hanburys.*

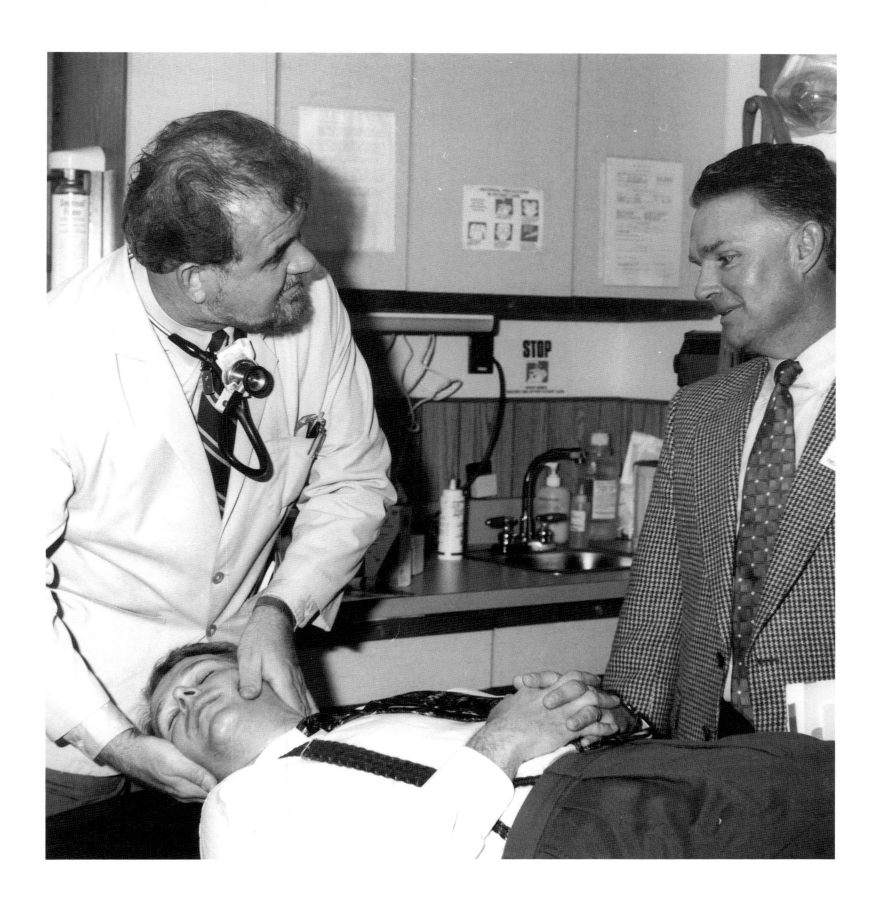

Although osteopathic physicians were not allowed to practice in the armed services during World War II, this discrimination proved to be a blessing in disguise. By proving their expertise on the homefront, in the absence of many allopathic physicians, osteopaths had the opportunity to serve as primary care physicians. As a result, the focus of osteopathy shifted from the treatment of chronic problems to broad-based care of patients.

Left: Two DOs deliver a baby in 1956 at the Chicago College of Osteopathic Medicine. Although not included in the original curriculum of osteopathic study, obstetrics eventually became an integral part of osteopathic primary care.

Right: Osteopathic and allopathic hospitals alike felt the effects of the post-WWII baby boom.

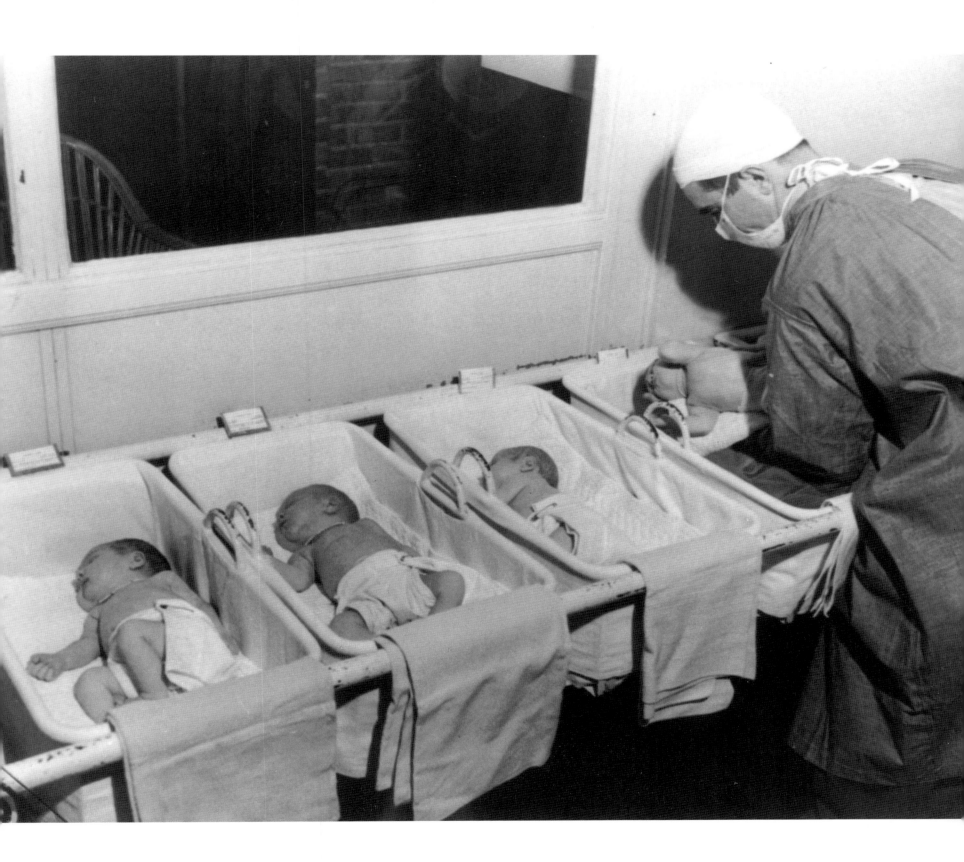

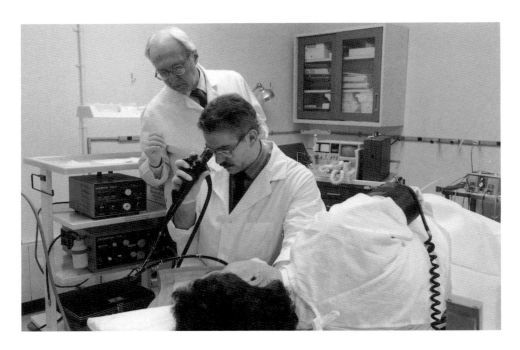

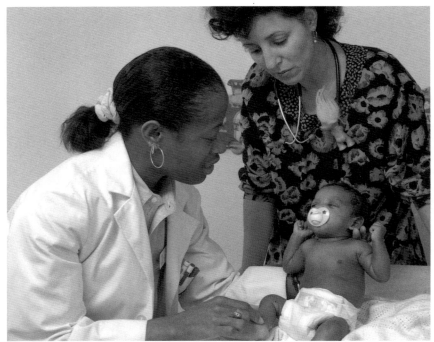

Above, top: *The judicious application of technology yields maternal-fetal health benefits in rural communities and urban areas alike.*

Above: *Over 55% of DOs practice in primary care specialties, including pediatrics.*

Right: *Each year 100 million patient visits are made to DOs in the United States.*

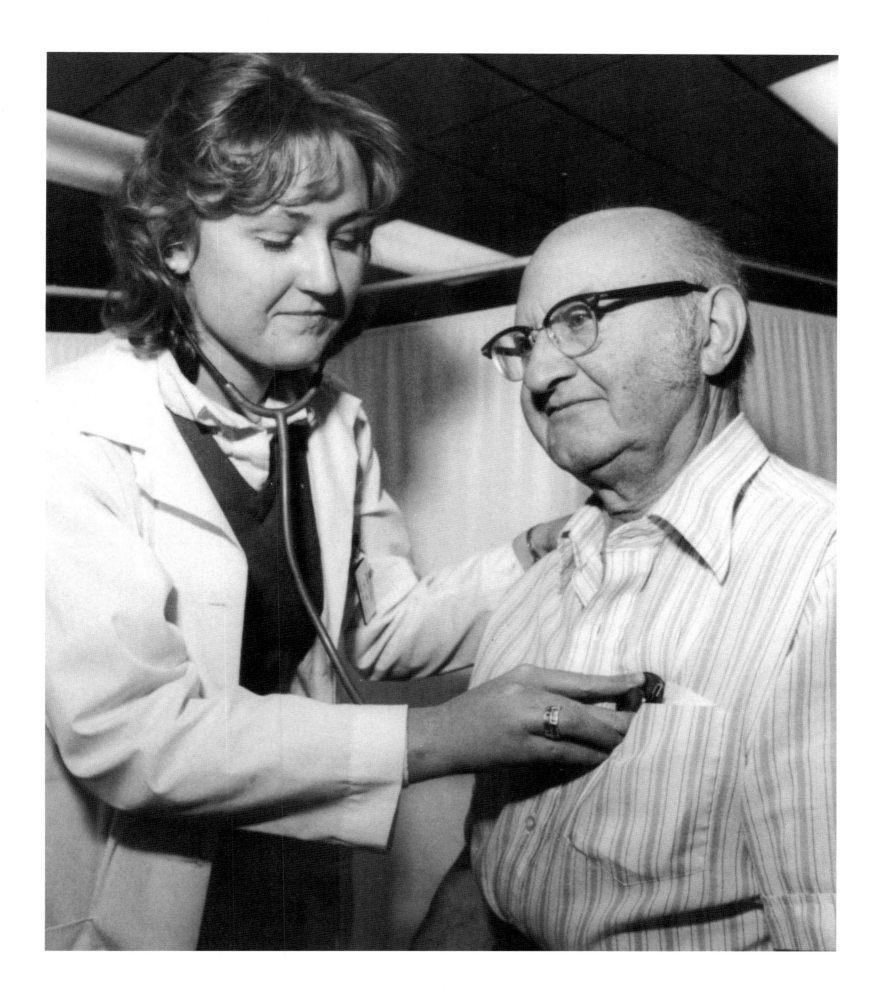

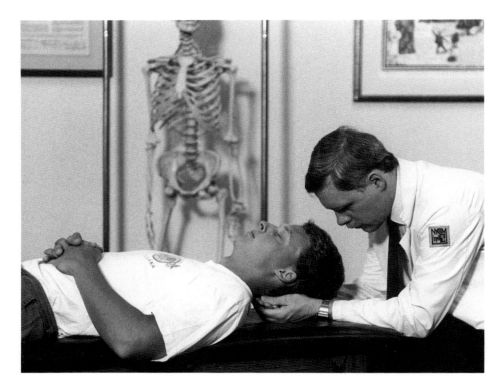

Above: *For a generation of DOs trained between 1940 and 1975, manipulative medicine fell into disuse as many of these physicians adopted the ways of their allopathic colleagues. However, more recently, studies have shown the effectiveness of osteopathic manipulative therapy (OMT). It decreases time and costs associated with hospital stays, and benefits patients with many medical problems. Once again, OMT has assumed a major role in the practice of osteopathic medicine.*

Right: *Osteopathic medicine with its focus on the musculoskeletal system is an ideal foundation for a career in sports medicine. The sports medicine program at the New York College of Osteopathic Medicine uses sophisticated technology like this CYBEX knee training equipment to help treat patients with knee injuries.*

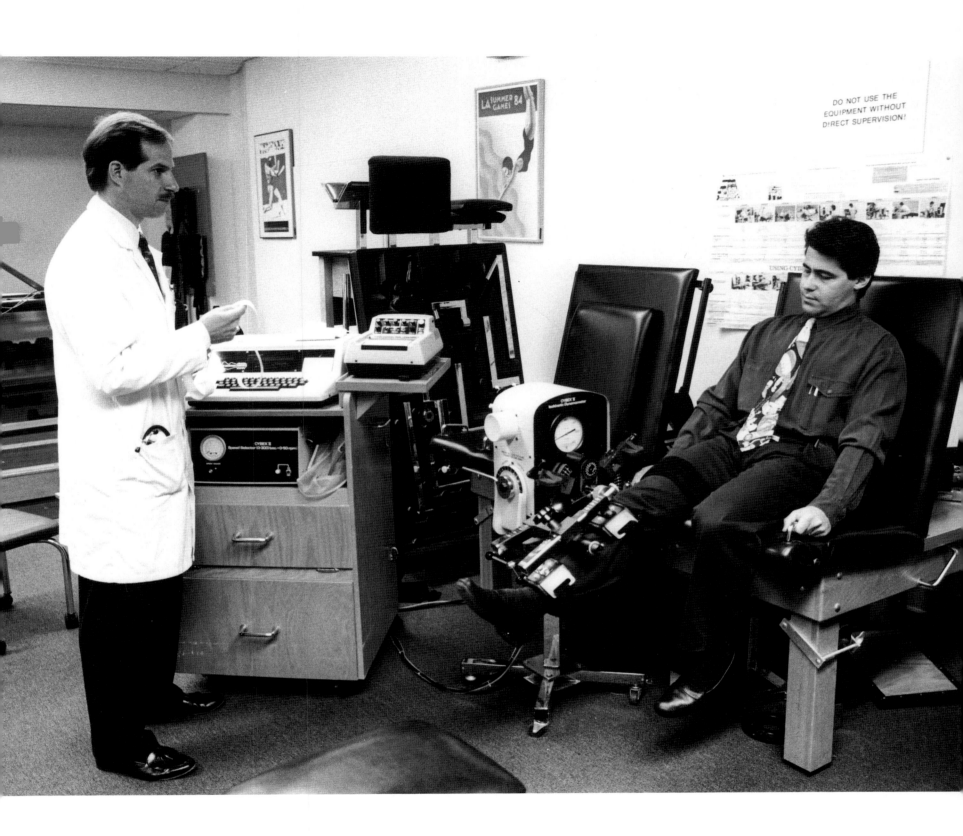

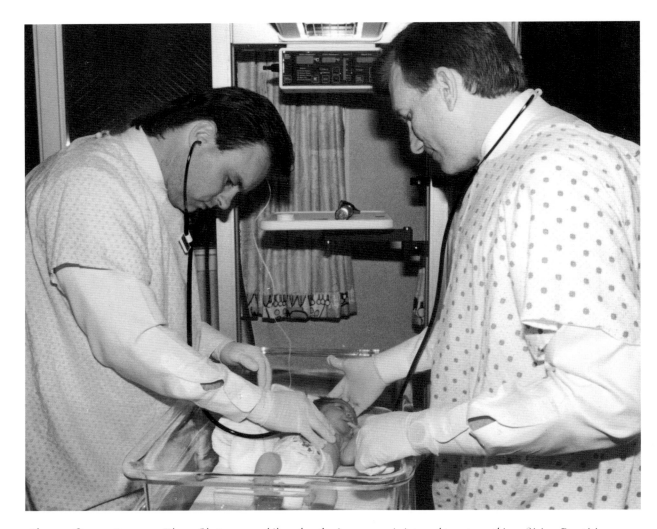

Above and opposite page: *The cradle-to-grave philosophy of primary care is integral to osteopathic medicine. Practitioners are taught that the value of touch goes beyond its diagnostic usefulness to also provide reassurance to patients of all ages.*

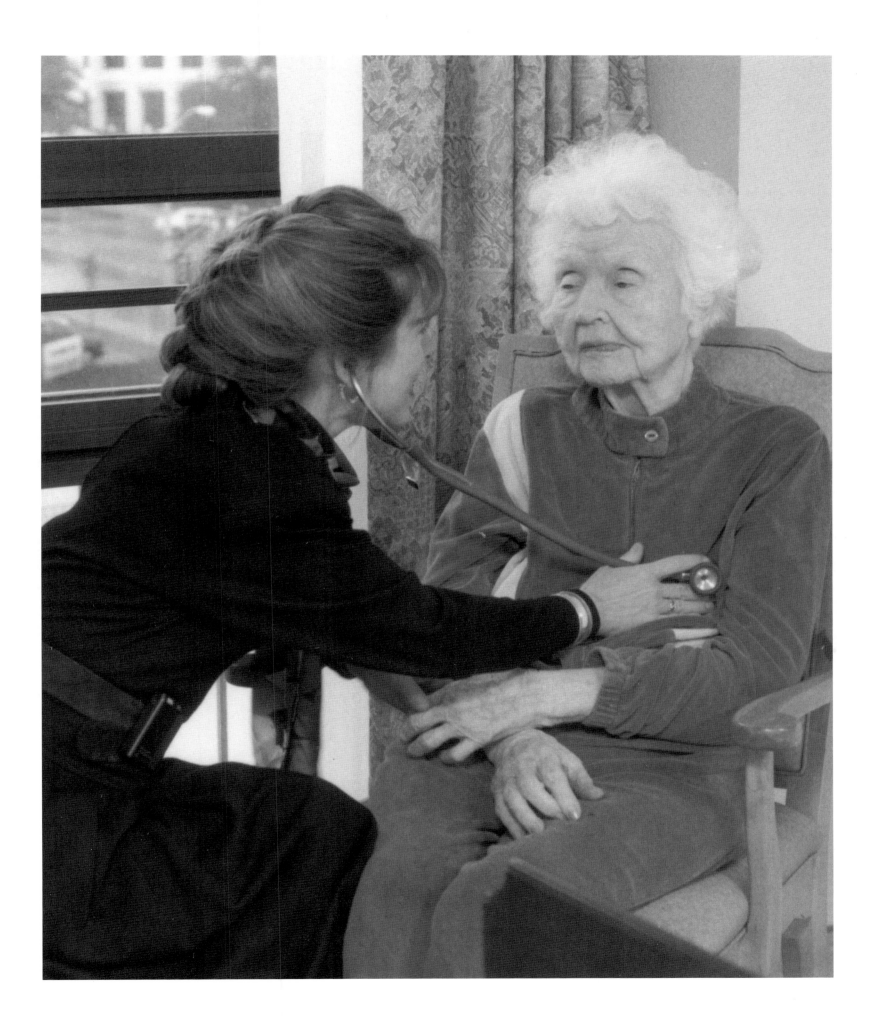

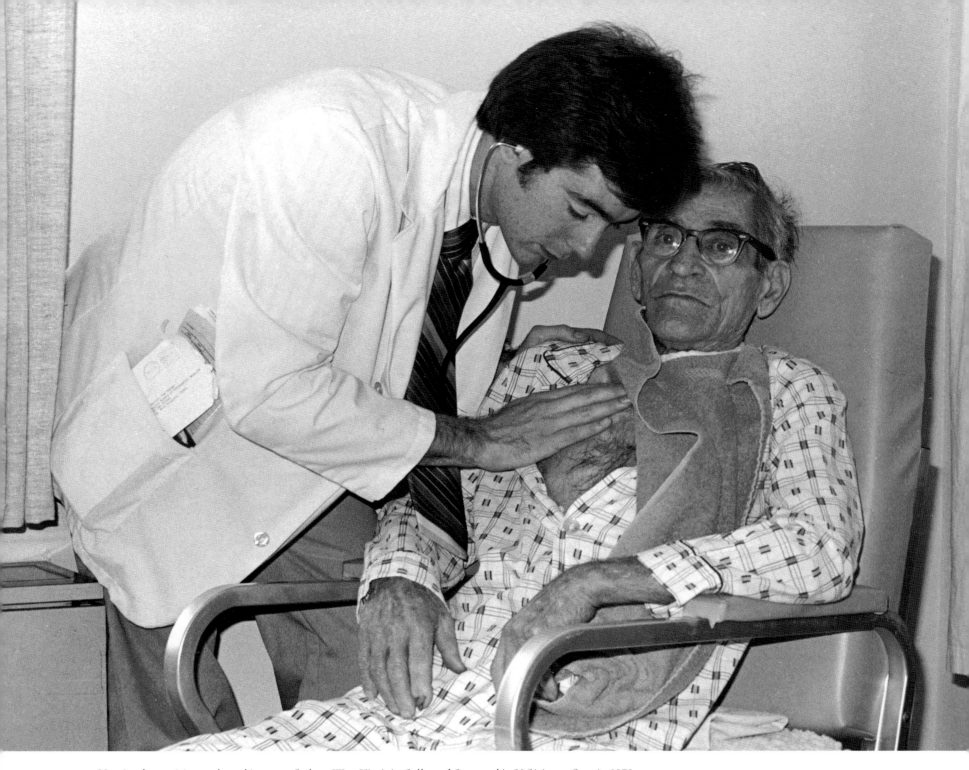

Nursing home visits, such as this one made by a West Virginia College of Osteopathic Medicine student in 1979, are becoming increasingly frequent as the population ages.

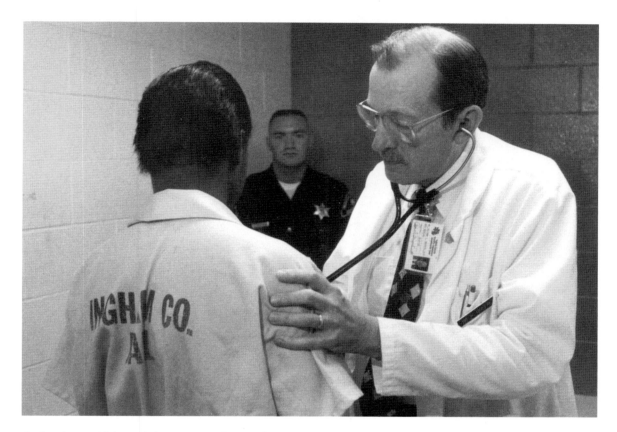

Under the watchful eye of the prison guard, a Michigan DO performs a health check on a prisoner.

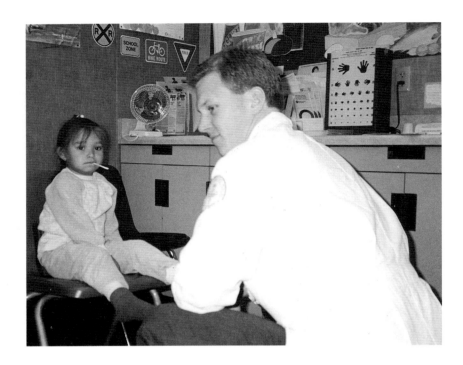

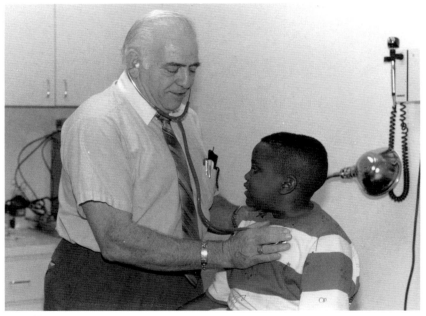

Above, top: *DOs participate in early childhood wellness programs such as the state-funded Healthy Start program in Pomona, Calif.*

Above: *Florida's Family Health Center and others like it at osteopathic medical schools throughout the country provide valuable medical services to the surrounding communities.*

Right: *Flu clinics for the elderly, such as this one conducted by the Ohio University College of Osteopathic Medicine, are another way DOs serve the health of their communities.*

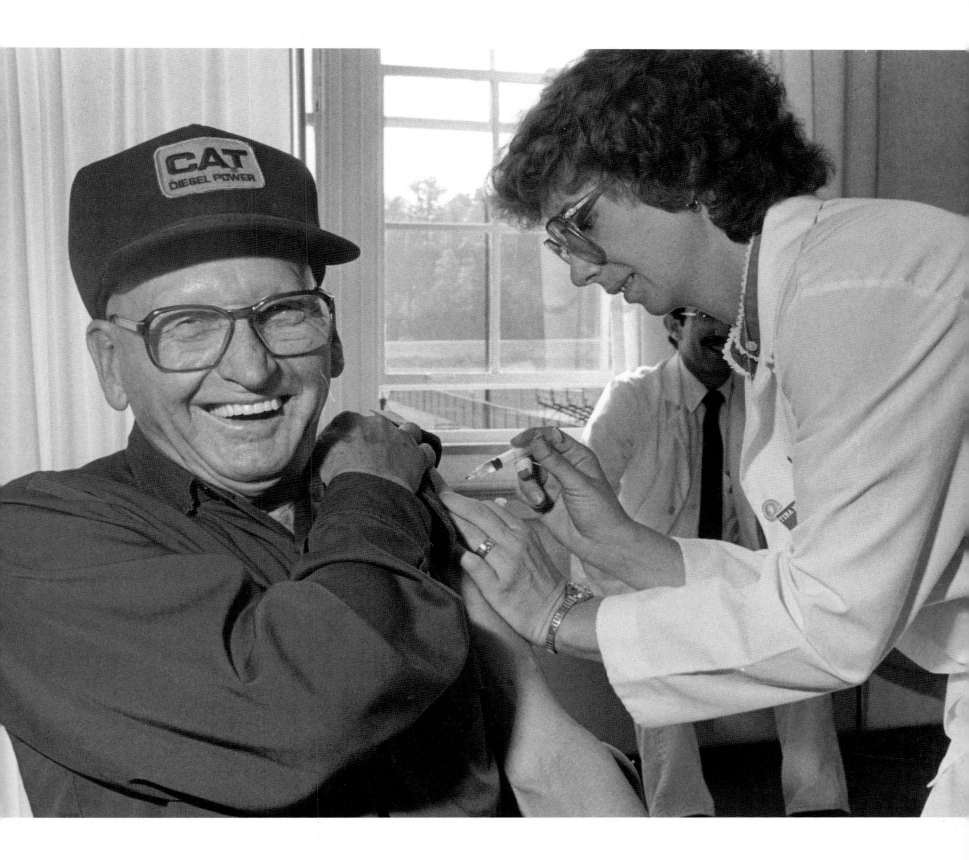

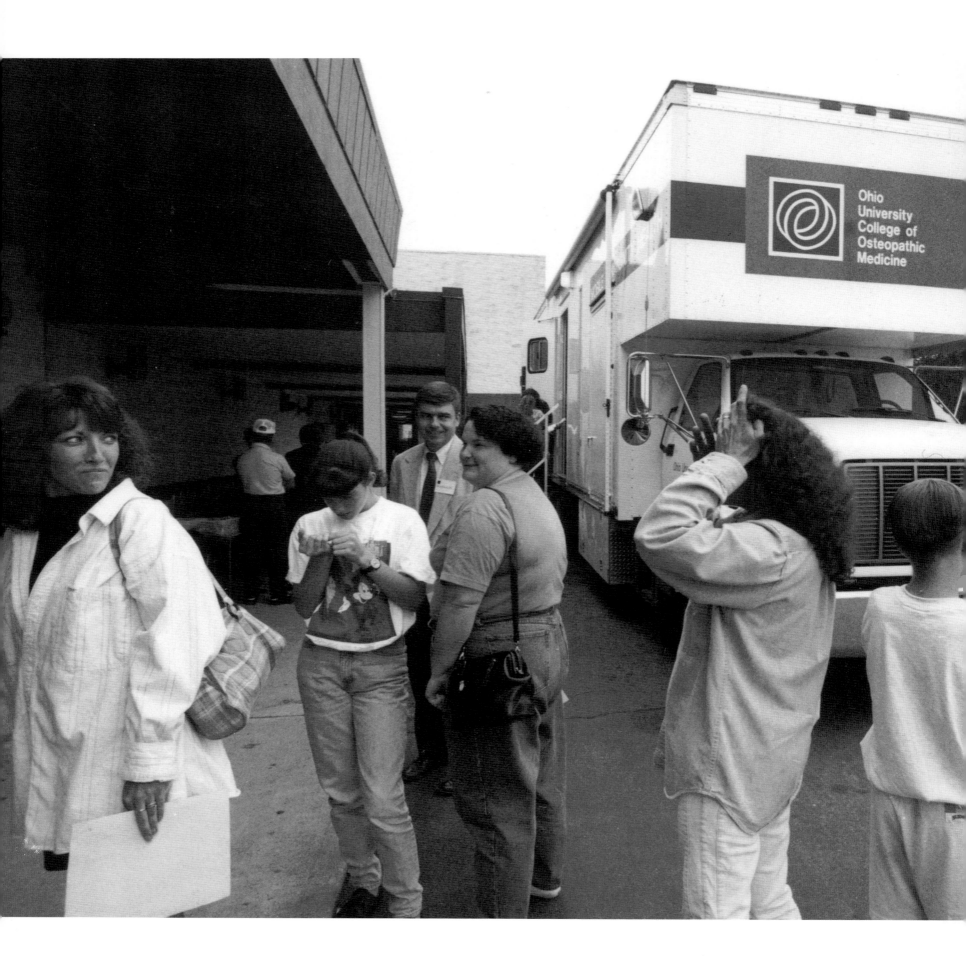

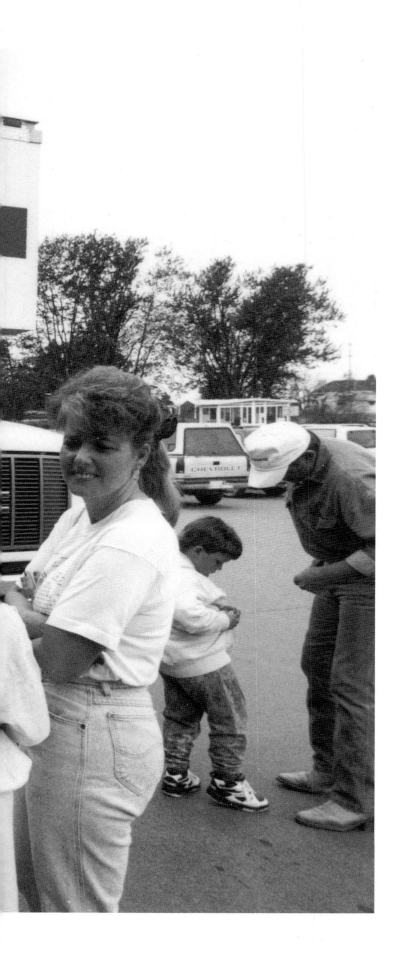

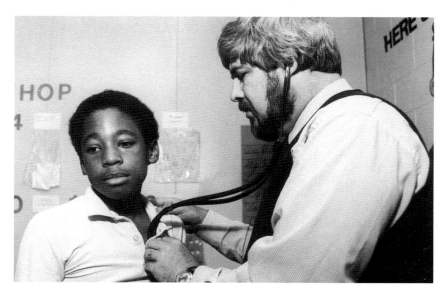

Left: Programs for early childhood health may include efforts to ensure immunization of all preschoolers, including sending a van into the community.

Above: The tradition of school-based health programs continues today and involves staff and students of the Michigan State University School of Osteopathic Medicine.

to learn and *To teach*

As the practice of osteopathy—and the number of schools that taught its principles—increased across the United States, the promulgation of accurate and scientific information became essential. In 1901 the *Journal of the American Osteopathic Association* was inaugurated by the AOA to facilitate the exchange of communication among its members and promote scientific knowledge. Shortly thereafter, rigorous standards were developed for the case studies that were included in their publications.

Clinical research to validate and advance osteopathic techniques received official support in 1913 when the AOA established the A.T. Still Research Institute in Chicago, Ill. Four years later, Louisa Burns, a graduate of Pacific College, headed up a West Coast branch, located near Los Angeles, Calif. The primary objective of this early research was to prove that visceral disease could be traced to "bony lesions" in the vertebrae.

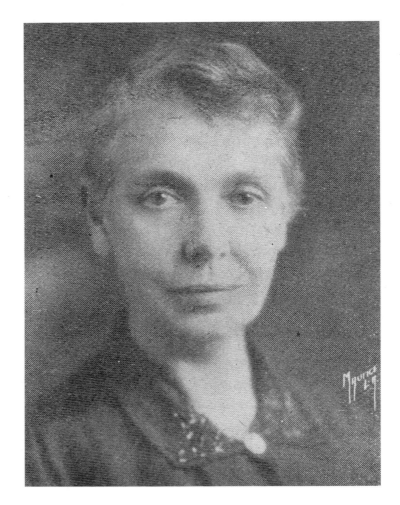

Right: *Louisa Burns, DO, was the first full-time investigator in in basic osteopathic research.*

Far right: *The Journal of Osteopathy, published monthly by the American School of Osteopathy, included anecdotal accounts of the remarkable cures effected by Dr Still. By 1897 its circulation list numbered more than 18,000 persons.*

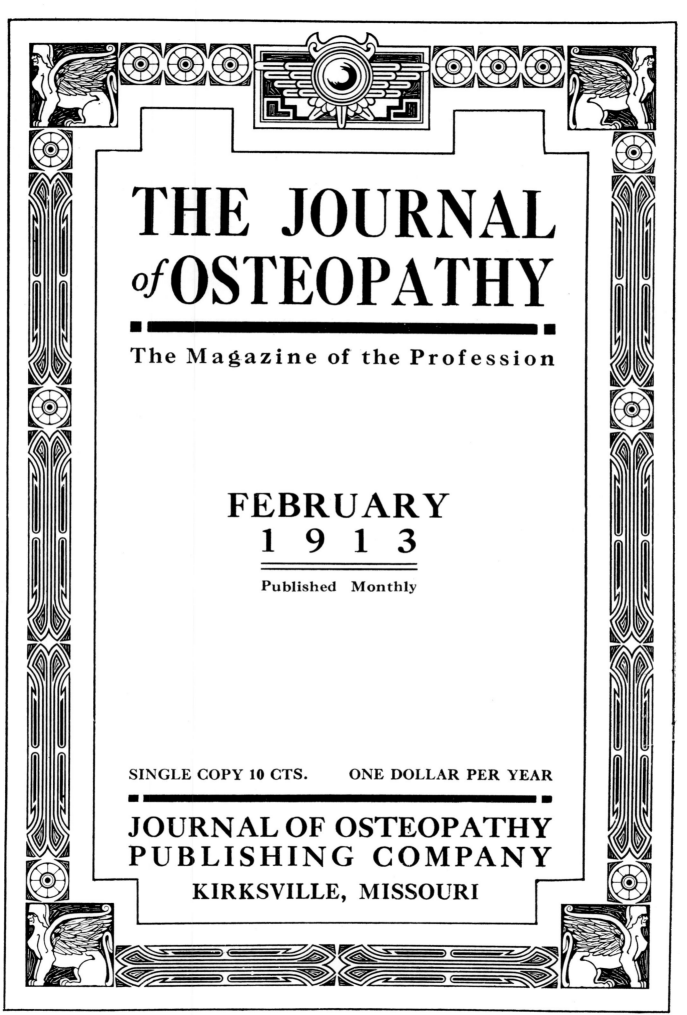

THE JOURNAL
of OSTEOPATHY

The Magazine of the Profession

FEBRUARY
1 9 1 3

Published   Monthly

SINGLE COPY 10 CTS.   ONE DOLLAR PER YEAR

JOURNAL OF OSTEOPATHY
PUBLISHING COMPANY
KIRKSVILLE, MISSOURI

With the development of electromyography, a new level of research on the role of the lesion was launched in the late 1930s. J. Stedman Denslow, DO, working with other researchers at the Kirksville College of Osteopathic Medicine, produced the first objective evidence of the existence of the lesion. In the early 1940s, several of their papers were the first reports of osteopathic research to be published in nonosteopathic journals.

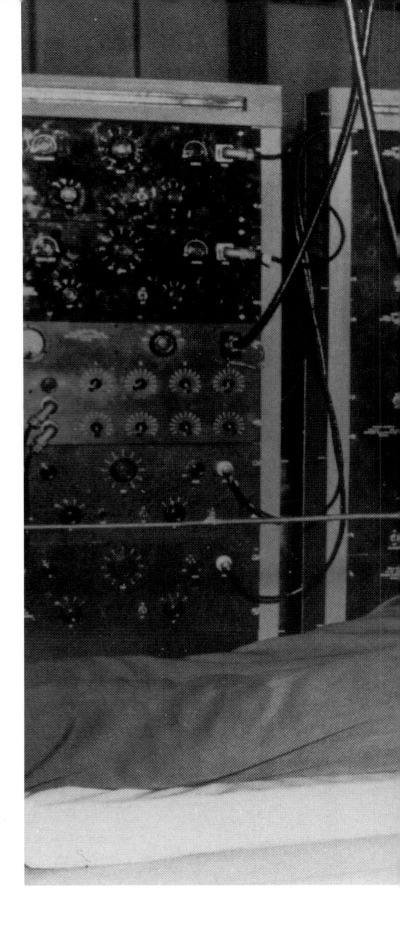

J. Stedman Denslow, DO, published the first report of osteopathic research in a nonosteopathic journal. Here the Kirksville researcher operates custom-designed equipment to verify palpatory findings in the 1950s.

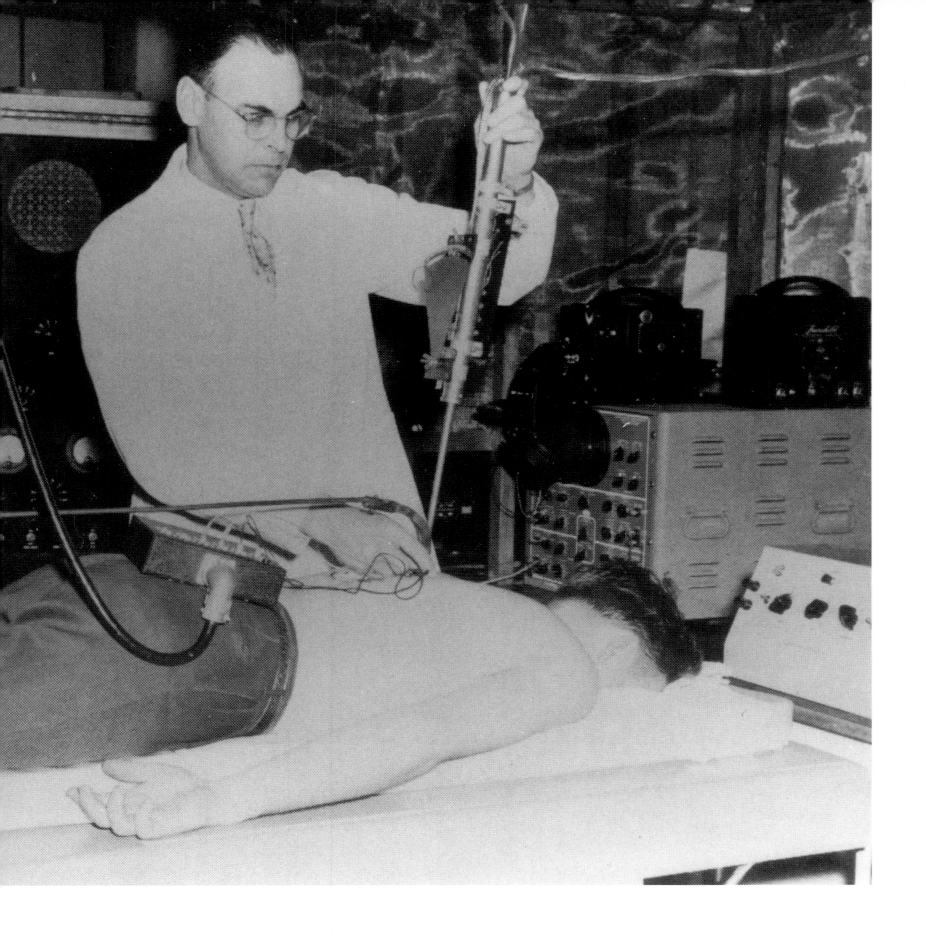

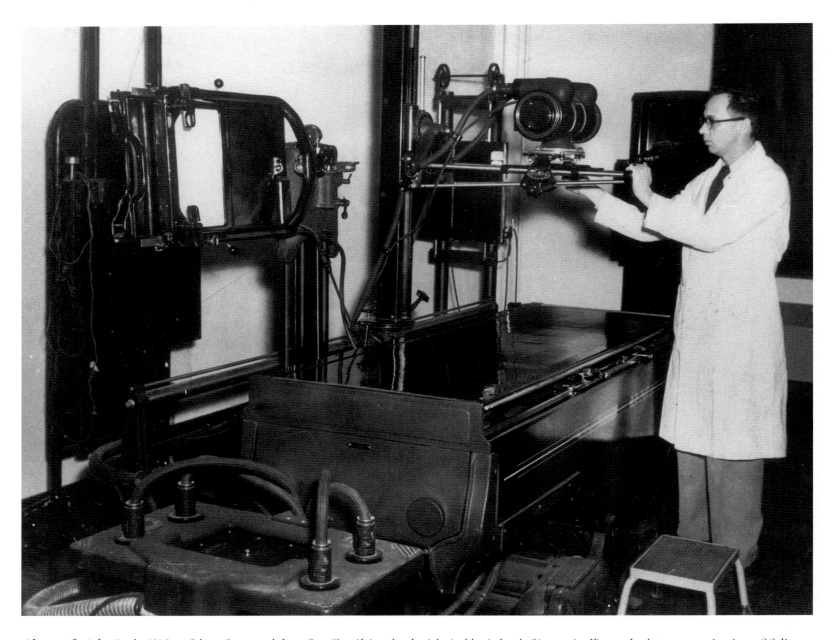

Above and right: *In the 1950s and beyond, research focused on identifying the physiological basis for the diagnostic efficacy of palpatory examination and delineating relevant physiological parameters that could be measured by electromyographic and other techniques.*

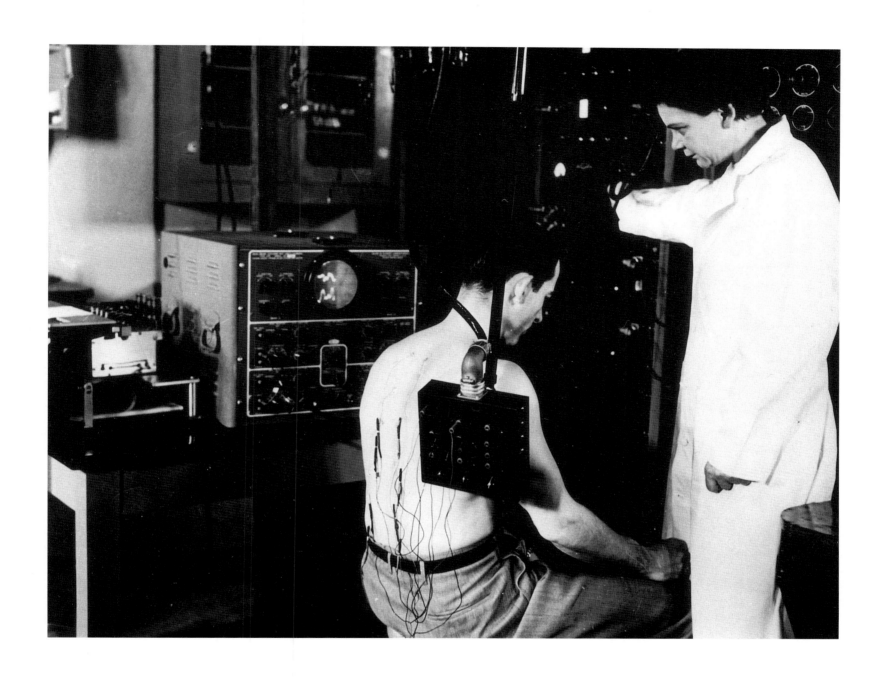

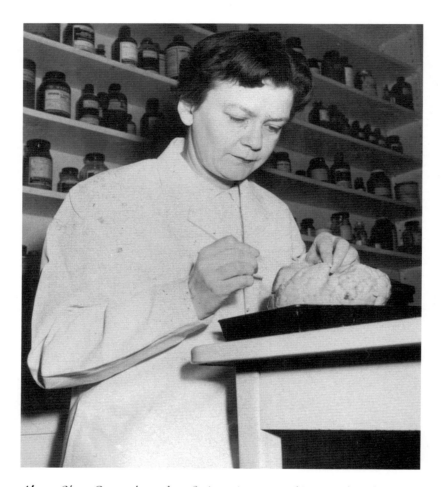

Above: *Olwen Gutensohn performed pioneering osteopathic research in the decades following World War II. An Australian by birth, she graduated from the Kirksville College of Osteopathic Medicine in 1959 and later taught a variety of medical courses there.*

Right: *Funding from the National Institutes of Health, state and local agencies, and private foundations enables modern-day osteopathic researchers such as Dr Arnold Hassen of the West Virginia School of Osteopathic Medicine to carry out research on a wide range of topics.*

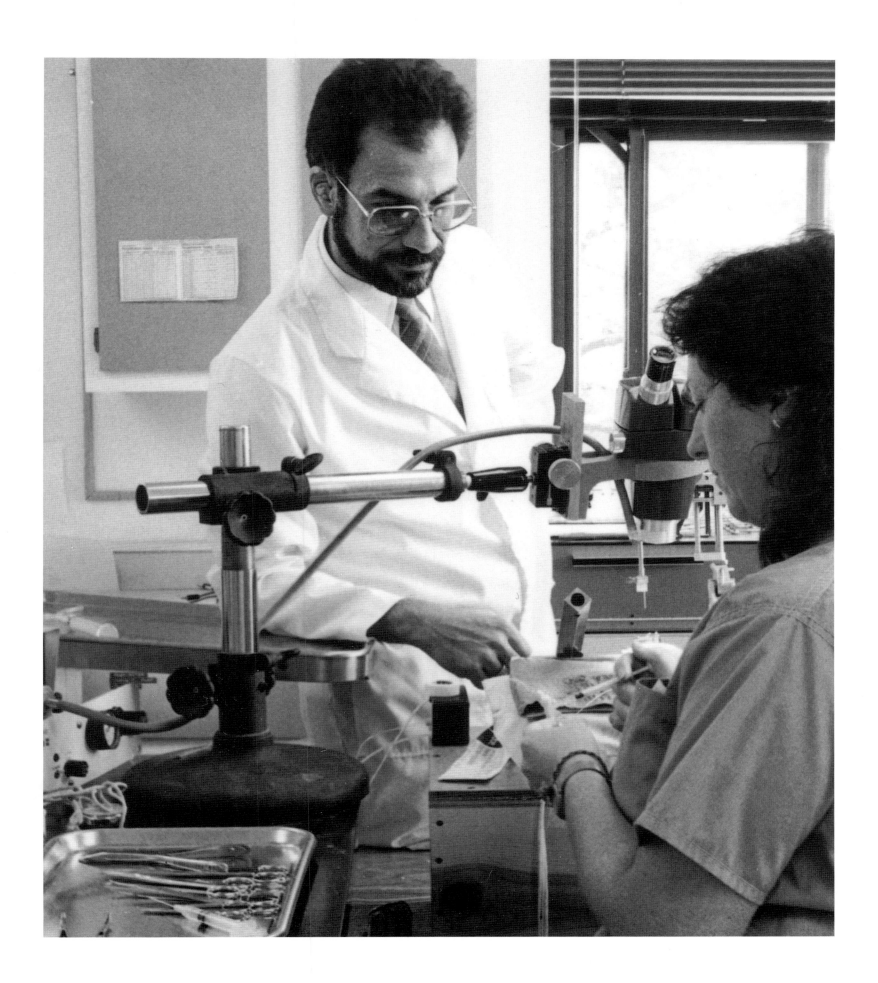

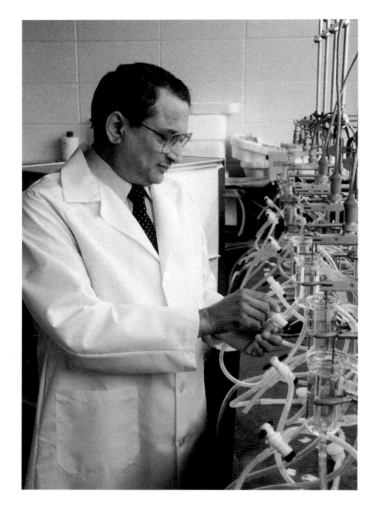

Above: *Dr Krishnakant Pandya joined the faculty at Kirksville as a pharmacologist in 1970. Today, his research efforts center on the tracheal and bronchial smooth muscle in the respiratory system.*

Right: *Researchers at the University of North Texas are directing their work toward finding cures for addiction, vision loss, osteoporosis, heart disease, and wounds that won't heal.*

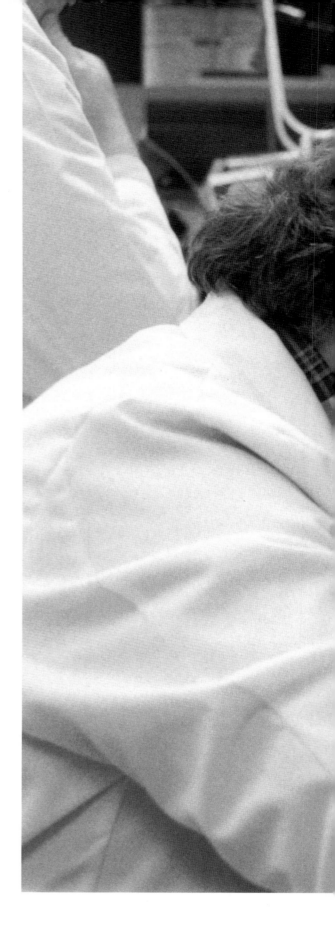

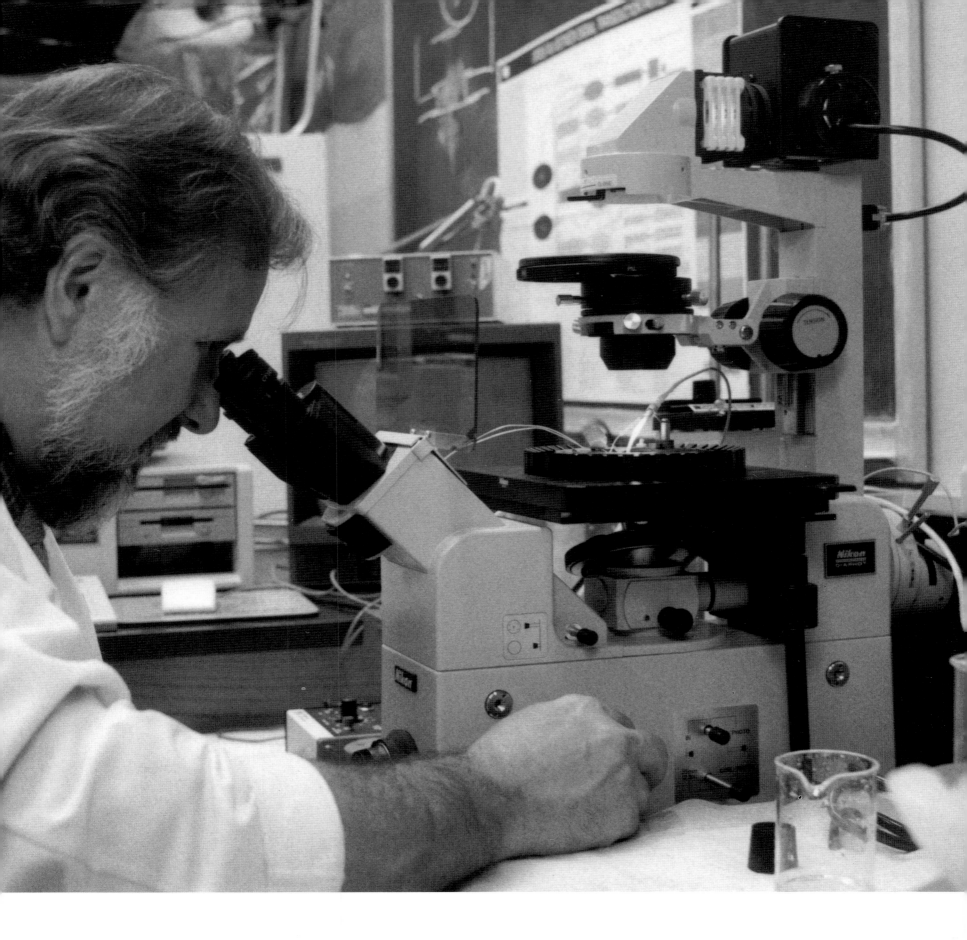

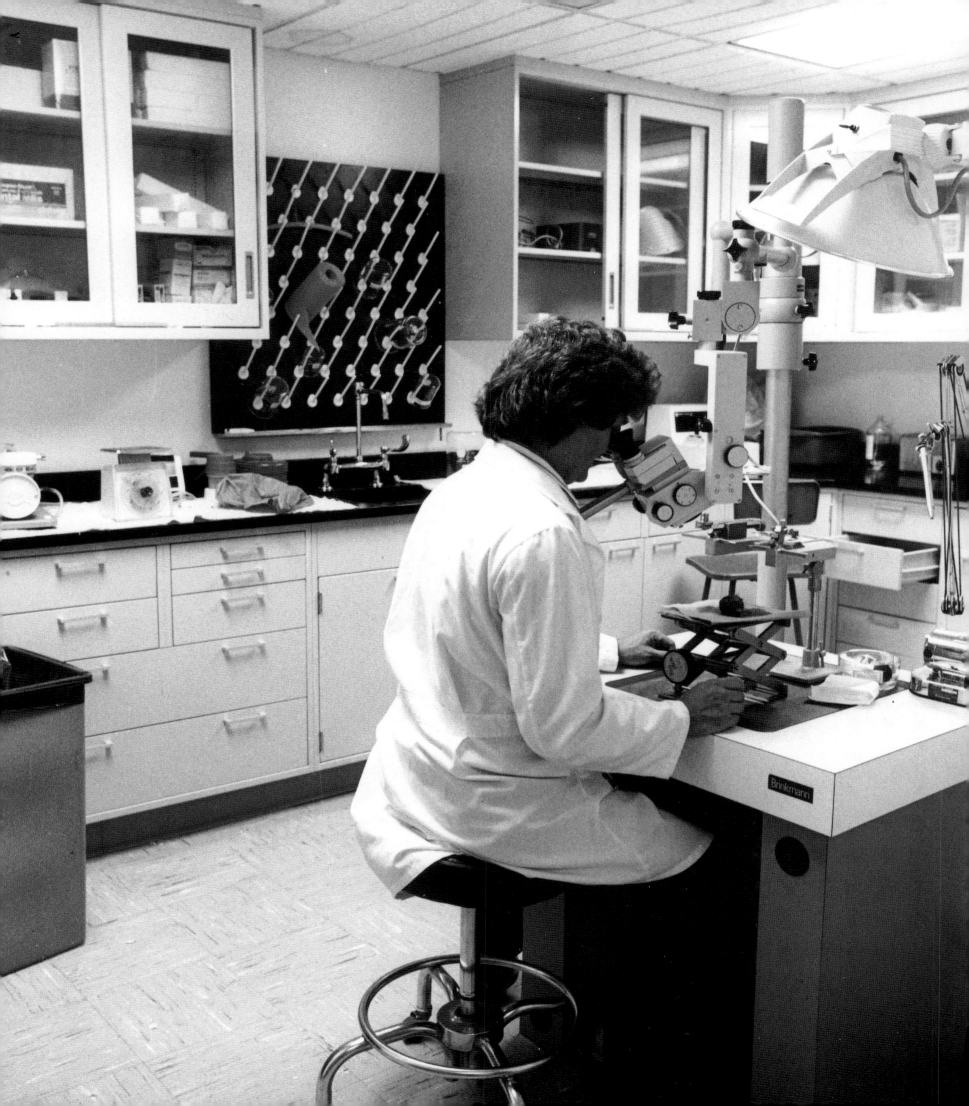

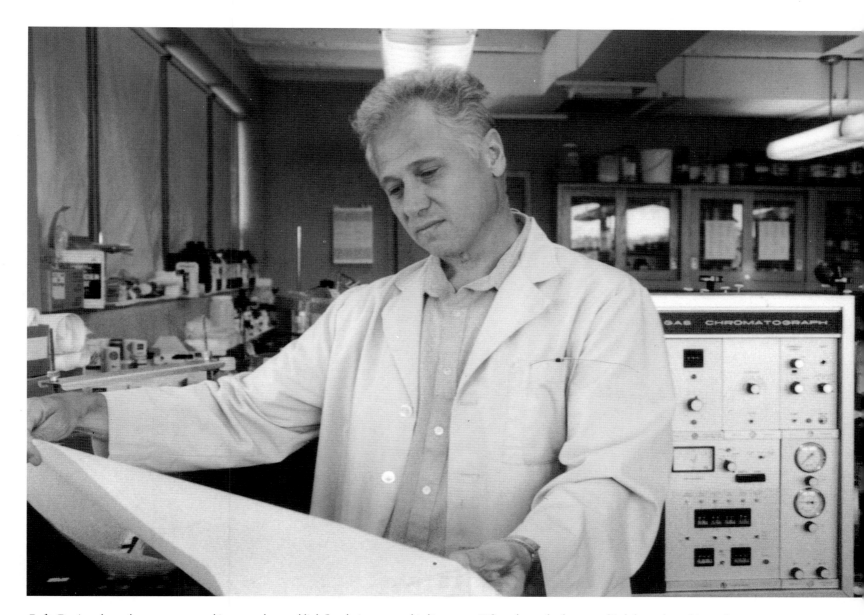

Left: *During the early years, osteopathic researchers published only in osteopathic literature. Today the work of osteopathic labs such as this one in New York appears in professional journals that represent every area of medical science.*

Above: *Dr Richard Cenedella performs biochemical research at Kirksville, specializing in studies of membrane biochemistry of the ocular lens. His lab has reported that depletion of membrane cholesterol results in permanent cataracts.*

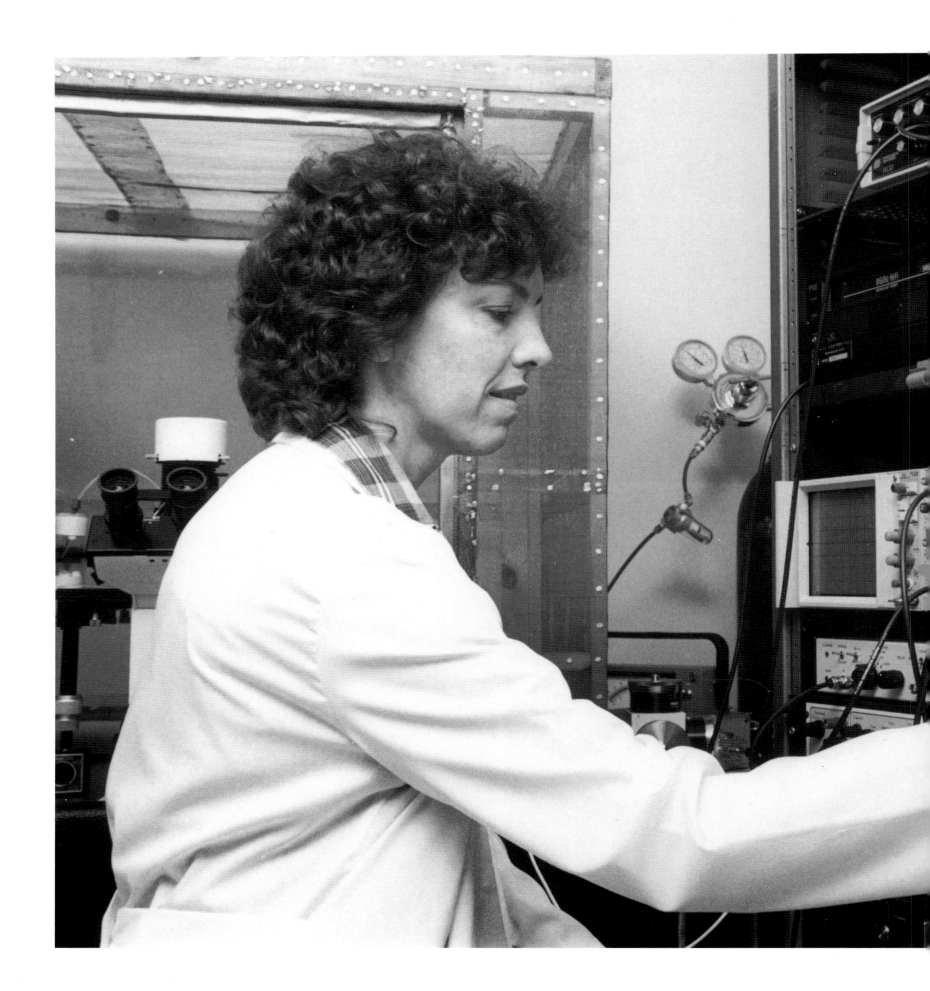

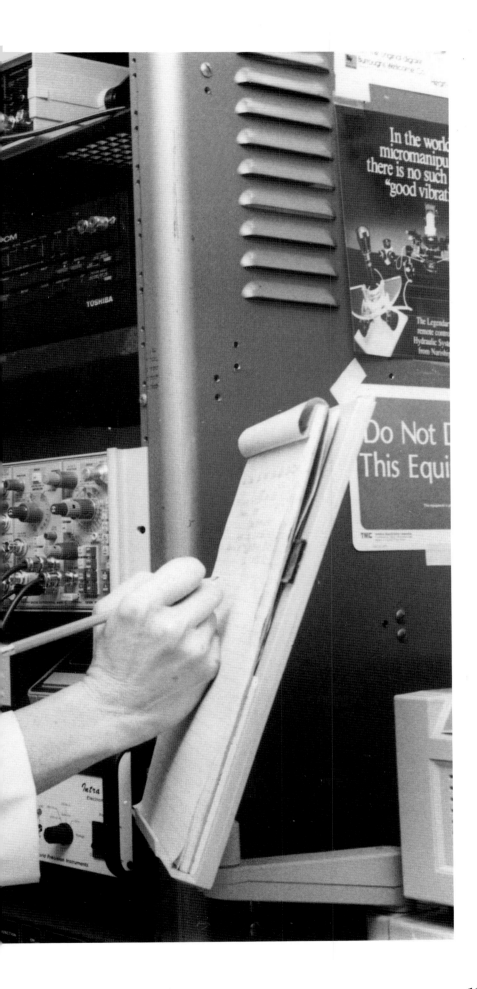

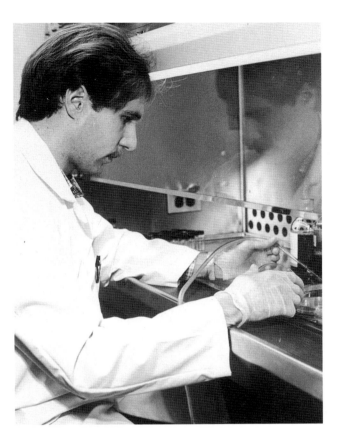

Left: *Kirksville researcher Dr Julia Ousterhout studies the pharmacology and physiology of vascular smooth muscle, including membrane electrophysiology.*

Above: *Scientists conduct osteopathic medical research in immunology, microbiology, pharmacology, anatomy, and physiology, exploring everything from genes to human organ systems.*

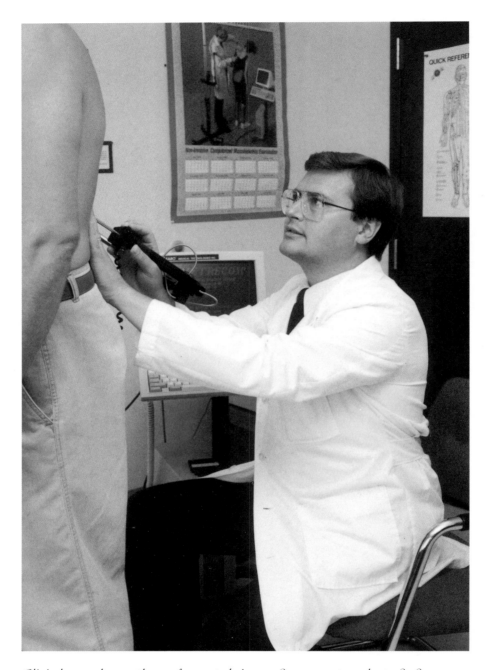

Clinical research paves the way for new techniques and new ways to apply standard therapies. For example, Dr Michael Kuchera at Kirksville has conducted numerous postural studies. His work currently centers on finding objective values related to pre- and postmanipulation measurements to demonstrate cost-effectiveness and clinical effectiveness of osteopathic manipulative therapy.

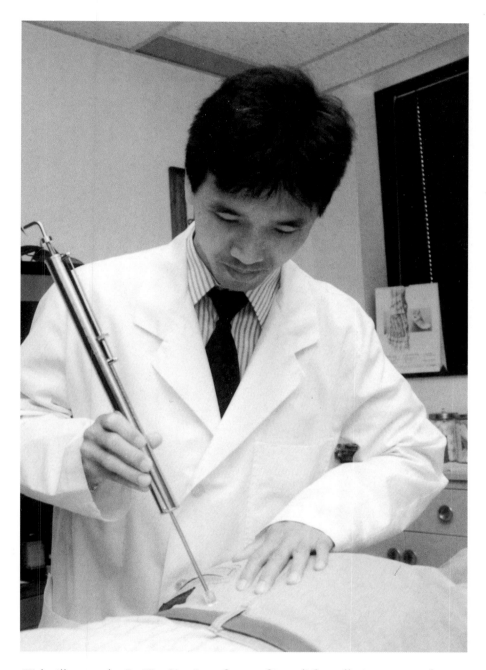

Kirksville researcher Dr Kim Sing Lo conducts studies to find an effective treatment for fibromyalgia in the spinal column.

The osteopathic curriculum of today demands dedication of faculty and students alike. The study of anatomy remains fundamental to an understanding of osteopathy. Although the sophistication of the science has increased, the precept that structure affects function has remained constant.

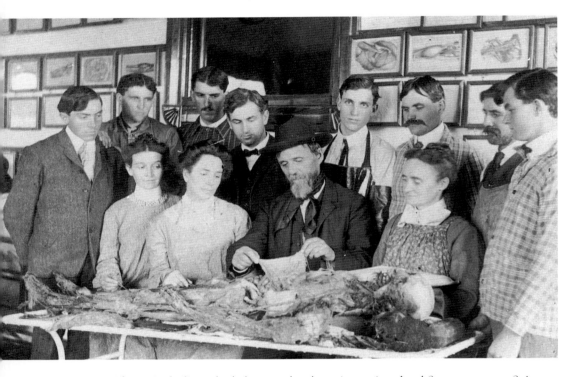

Above: *At the first school of osteopathy, the major portion of each day was spent studying anatomy under the tutelage of A. T. Still or his faculty.*

Right: *From the very beginning of osteopathic medicine through today, anatomy remains at the core of preclinical training. Here an instructor of anatomy uses models to teach fundamentals in 1952 at Philadelphia College of Osteopathy.*

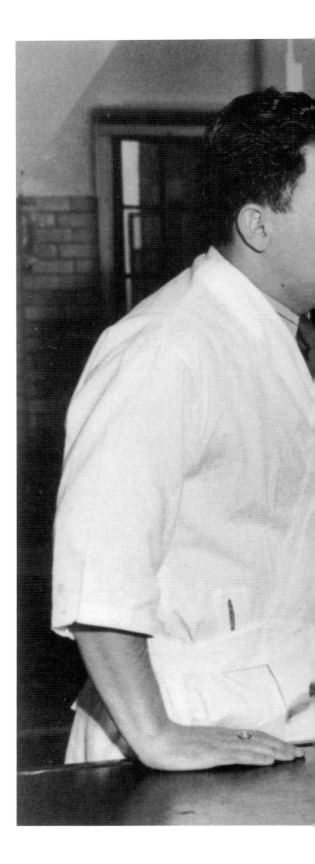

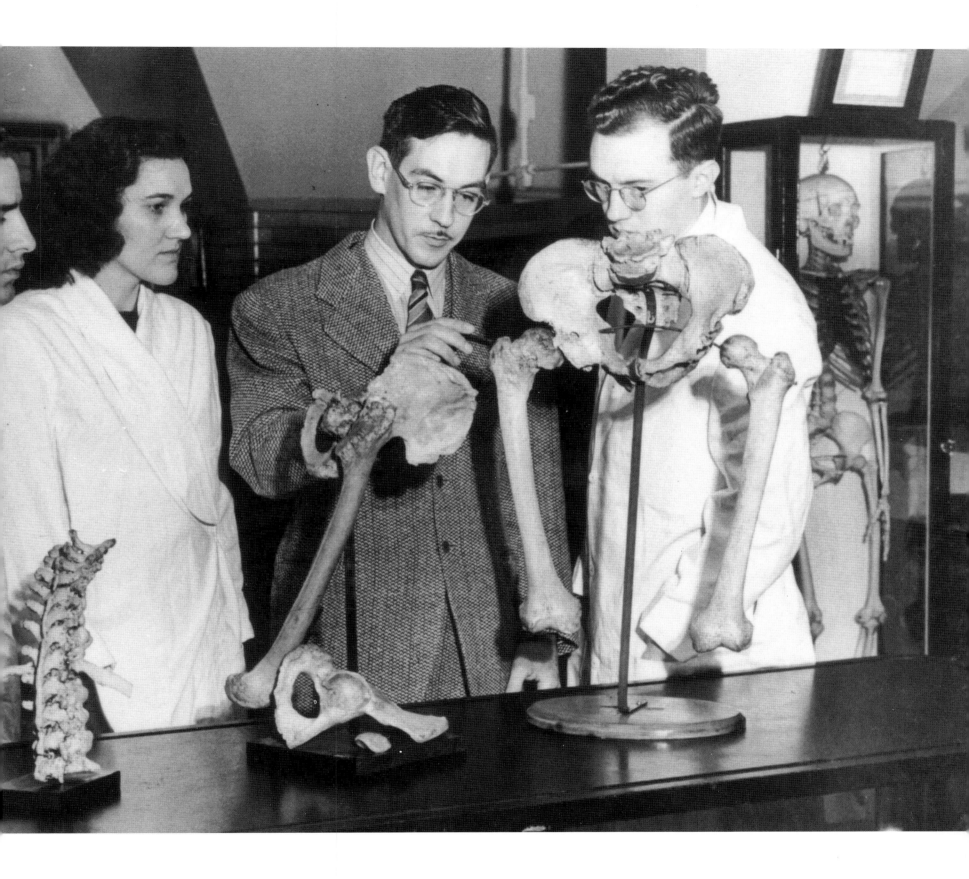

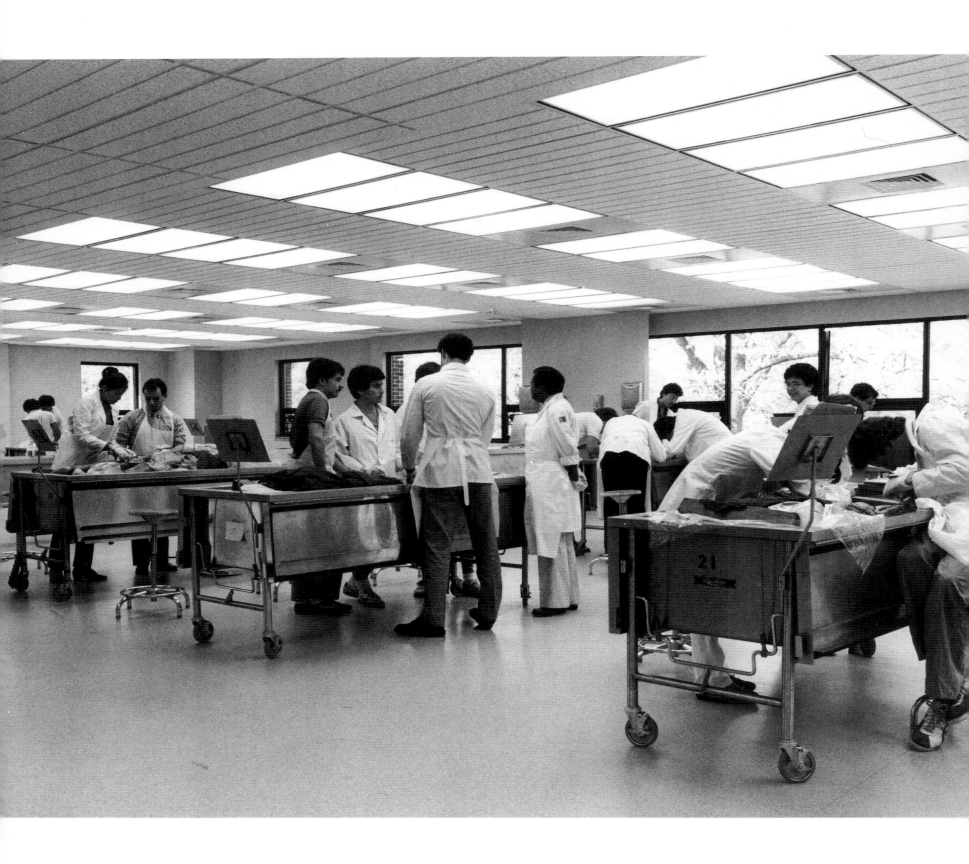

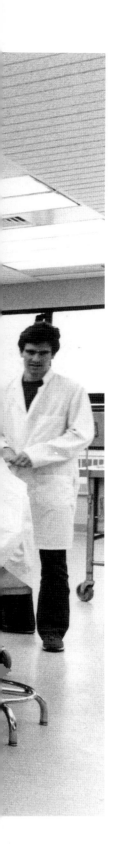

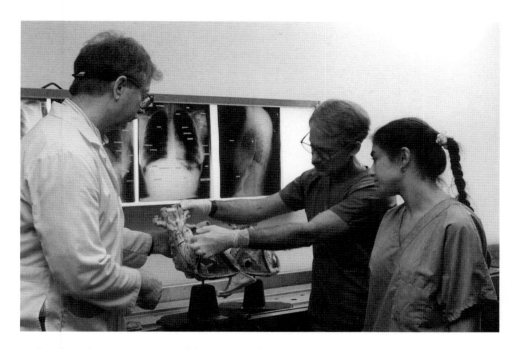

Left: The modern gross anatomy laboratory, such as this one in New York, is far removed from that at Kirksville at the turn of the century, but its fundamental value to the osteopathic student remains unchanged.

Above: Modern anatomical instruction makes use of models, radiographs, and other techniques to teach this fundamental subject.

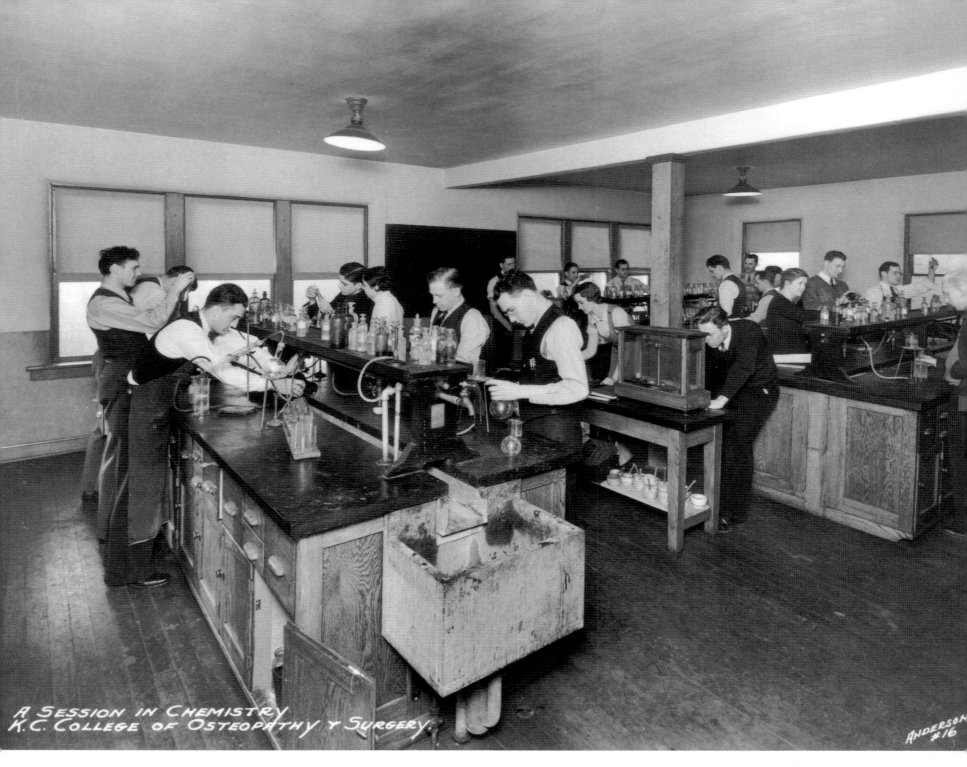

From the mid-1930s onward, the percentage of time spent in laboratories versus lecture halls during preclinical training rose significantly, with a 10% increase between 1935 and 1948 alone.

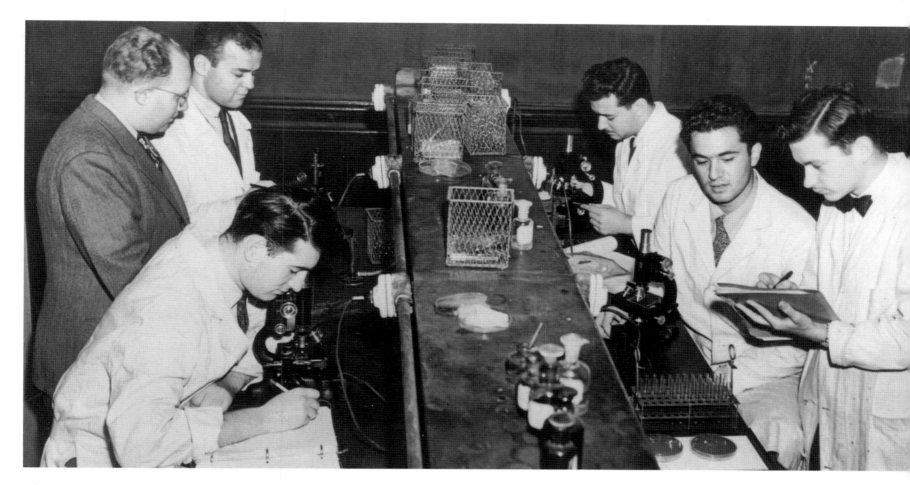

Above and overleaf: *Preclinical laboratory training included pathology, microbiology, biochemistry, anatomy, and physiology.*

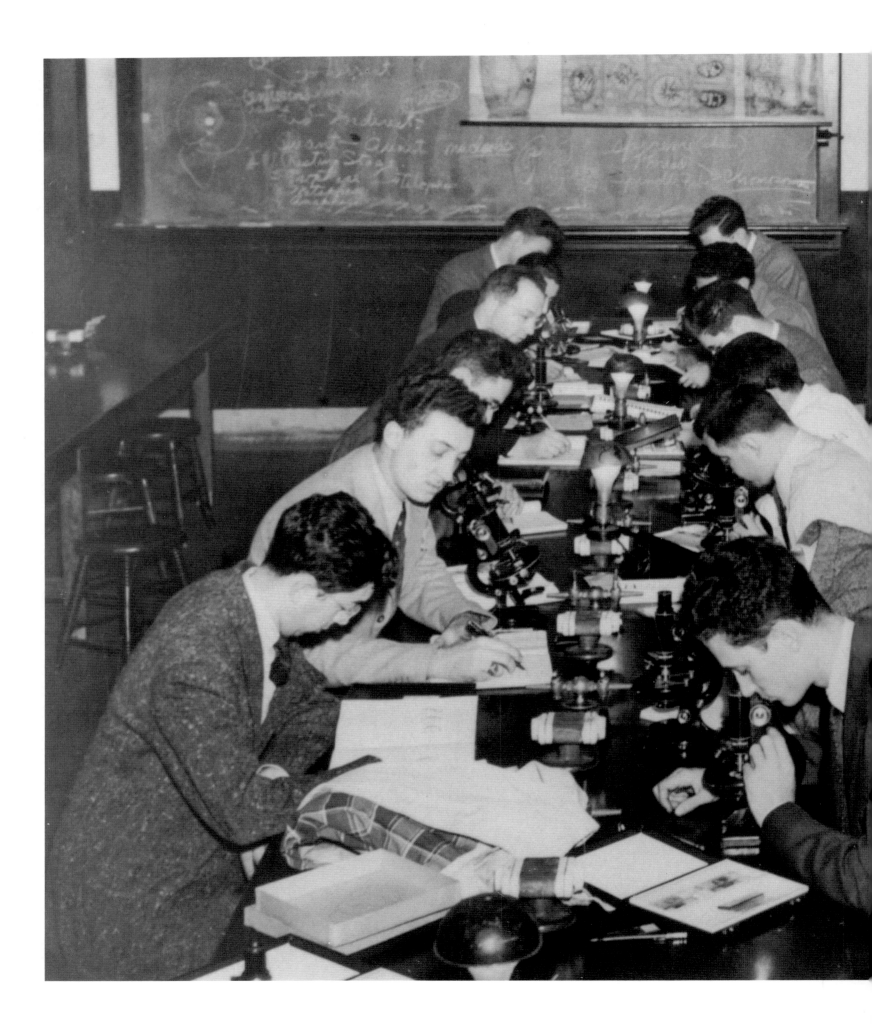

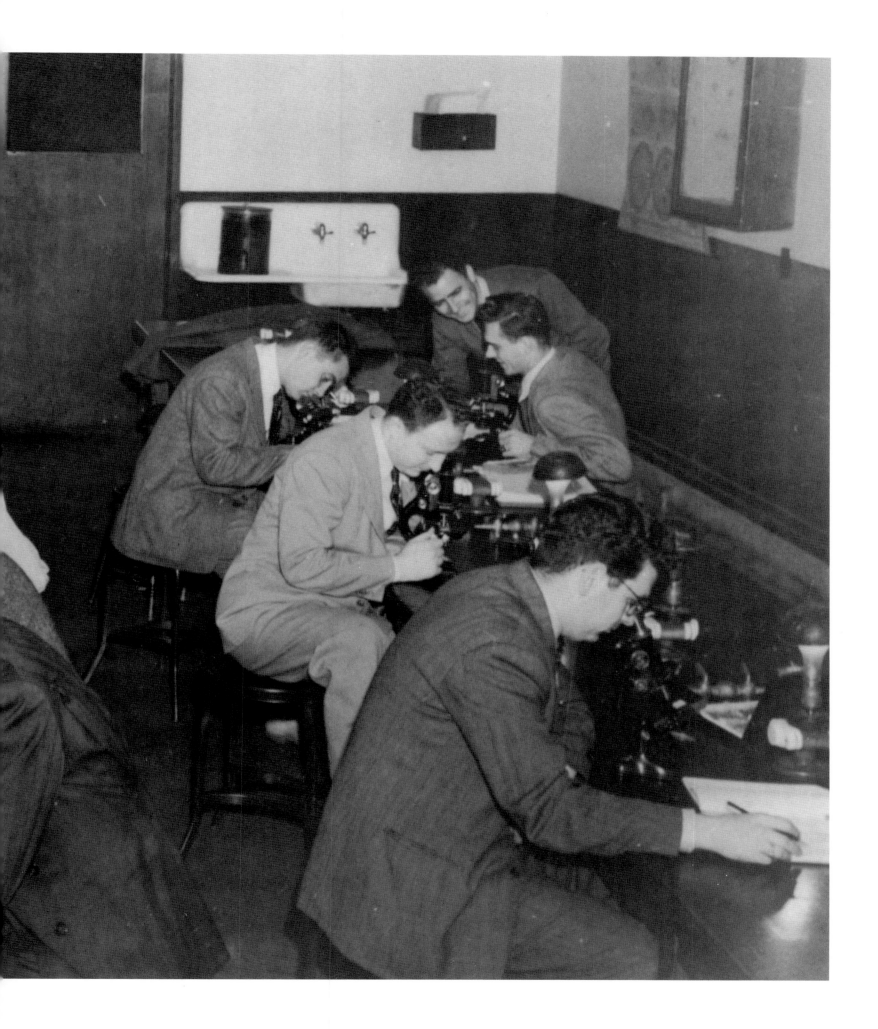

An histology laboratory at the New York College of Osteopathic Medicine.

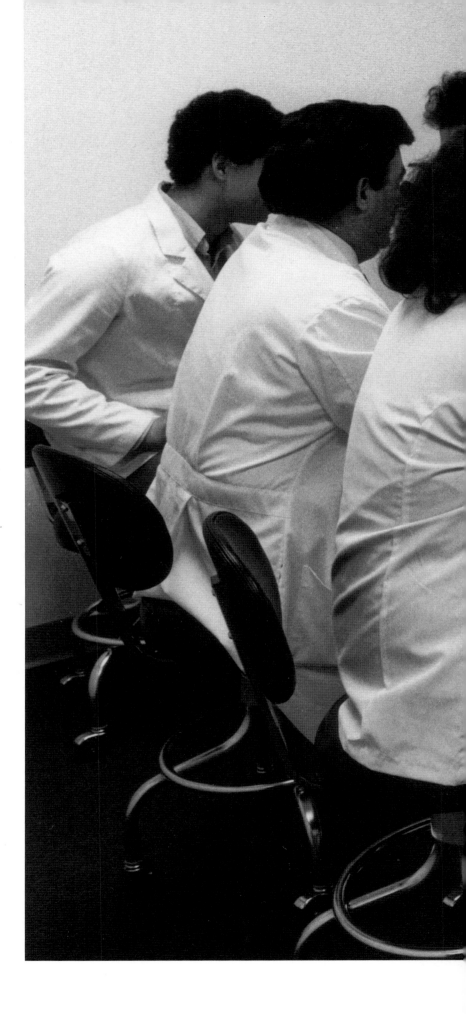

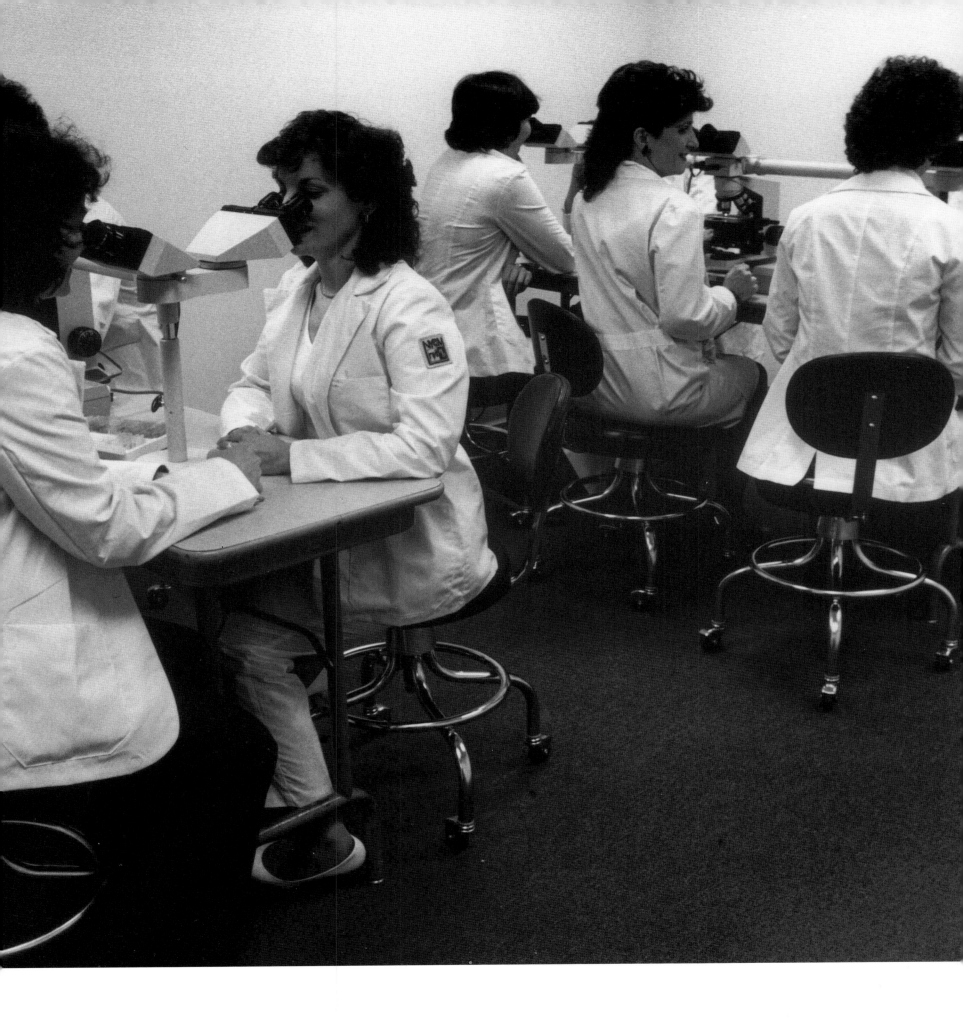

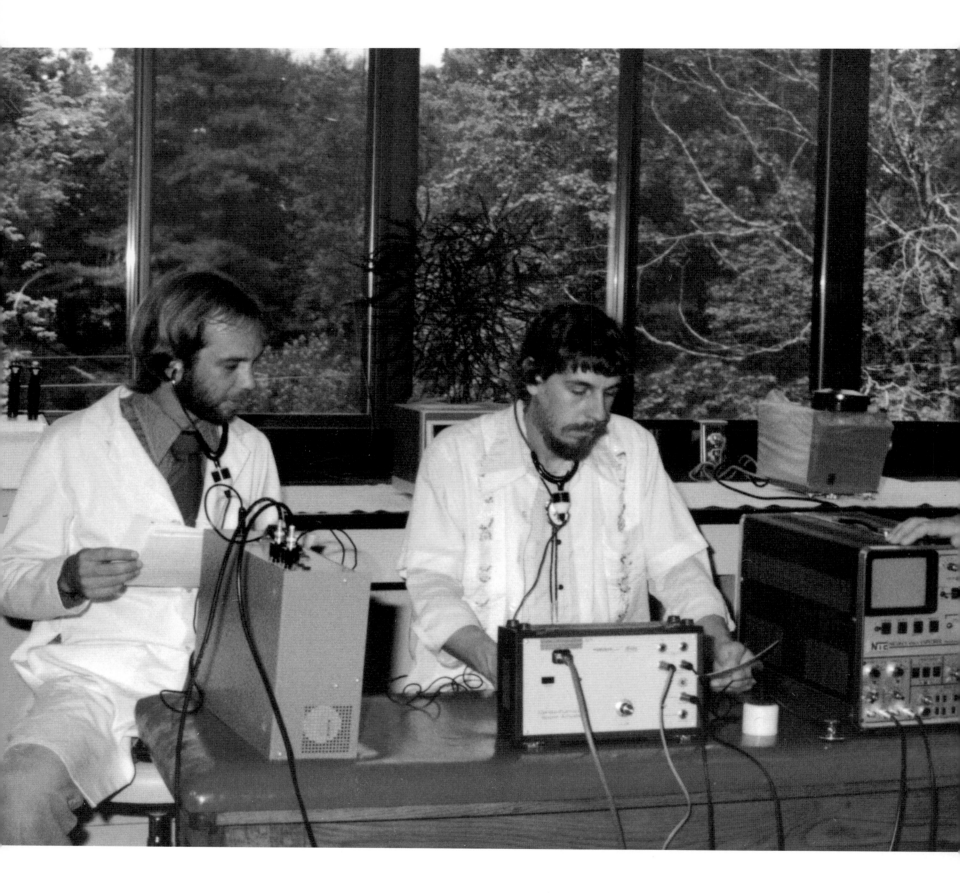

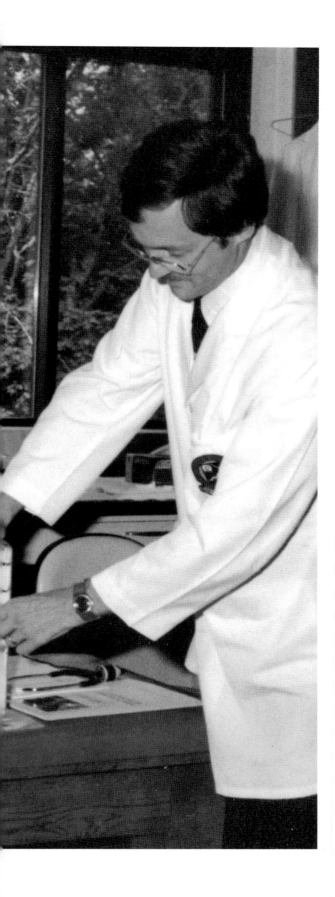

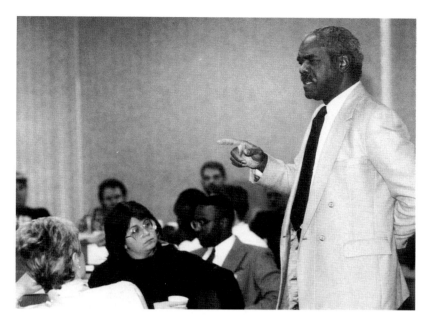

Left: *The oscillation laboratory, shown here at West Virginia circa 1980, is also a part of the osteopathic medical student's preclinical education.*

Above: *Visits to the classroom by practicing DOs help provide a patient-based reality to early studies during the preclinical phase.*

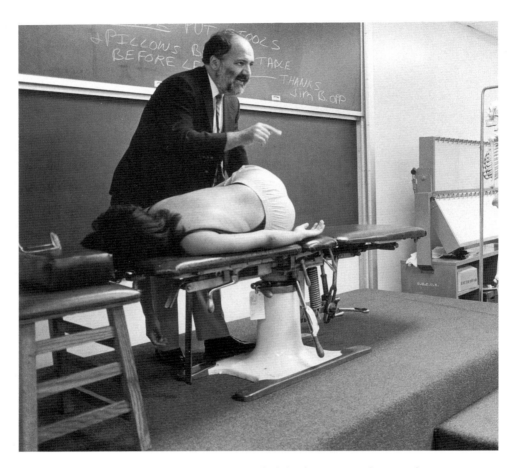

Above: *Dr Anthony Chua gives a lesson in musculoskeletal anatomy and manipulation.*

Right: *Instructors make use of every tool at hand, including their own bodies, to help students visualize key concepts of body mechanics.*

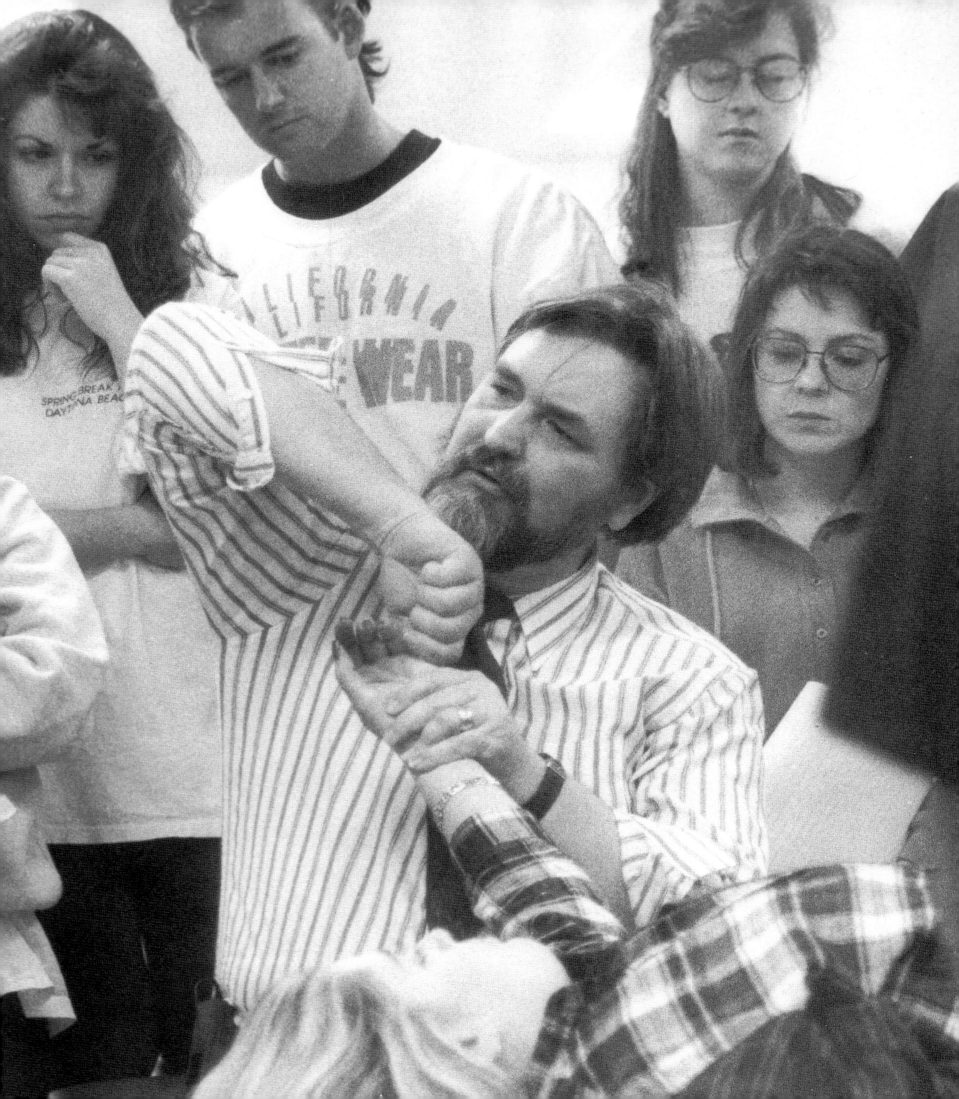

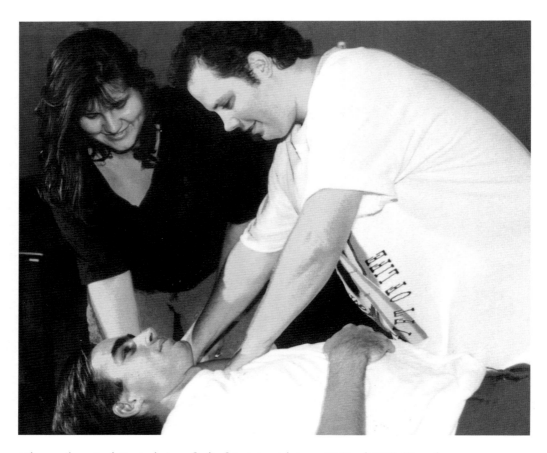

The use of manipulative techniques declined in interest between 1940 and 1970. Since then, however, manipulation has achieved renewed acceptance and a resurgence in current practice, research, and education. As with other techniques of patient care, the students must practice musculoskeletal manipulation to attain proficiency.

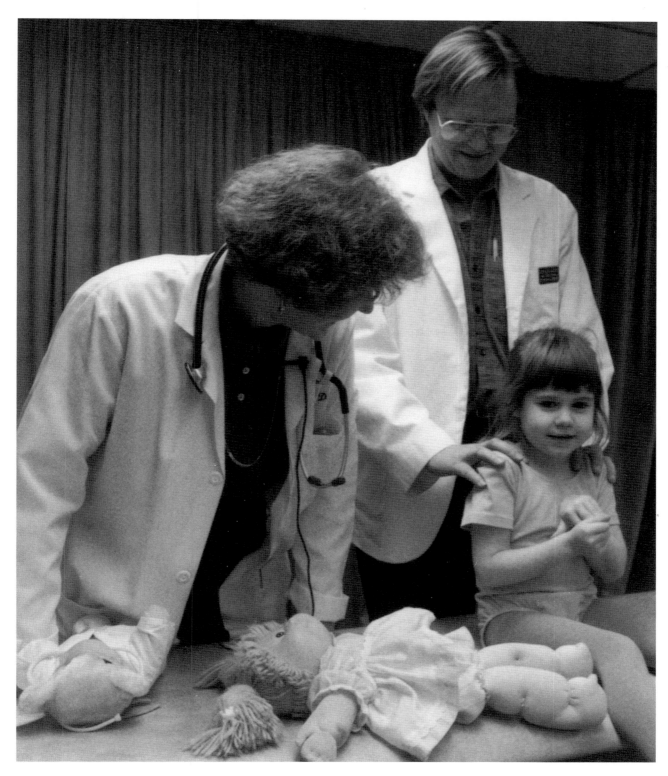

Patient volunteers in the classroom help osteopathic students hone their interpersonal and communication skills.

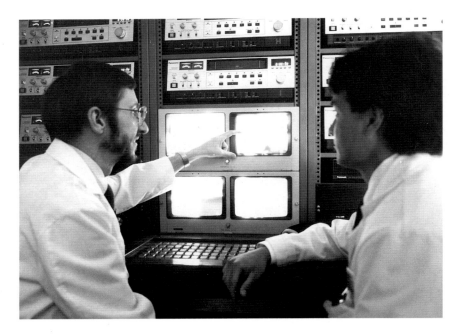

Above: With its emphasis on patient-centered medicine, osteopathic medicine takes advantage of every available tool in training its students for patient care, such as this videotaped patient simulation program at Ohio University.

Right: Clinical training continually reminds students of the importance of the musculoskeletal system.

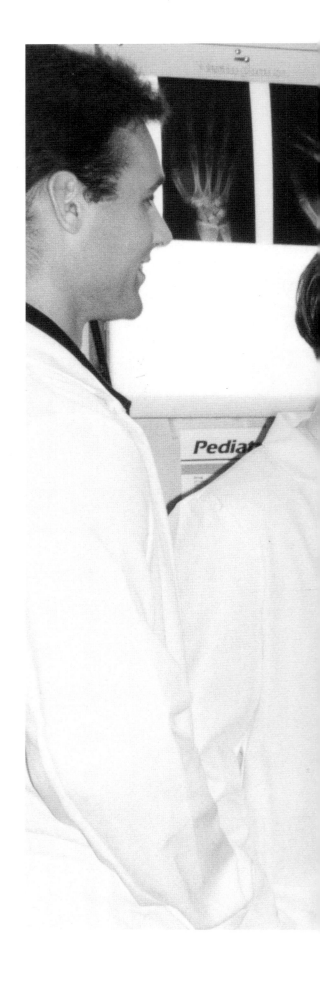

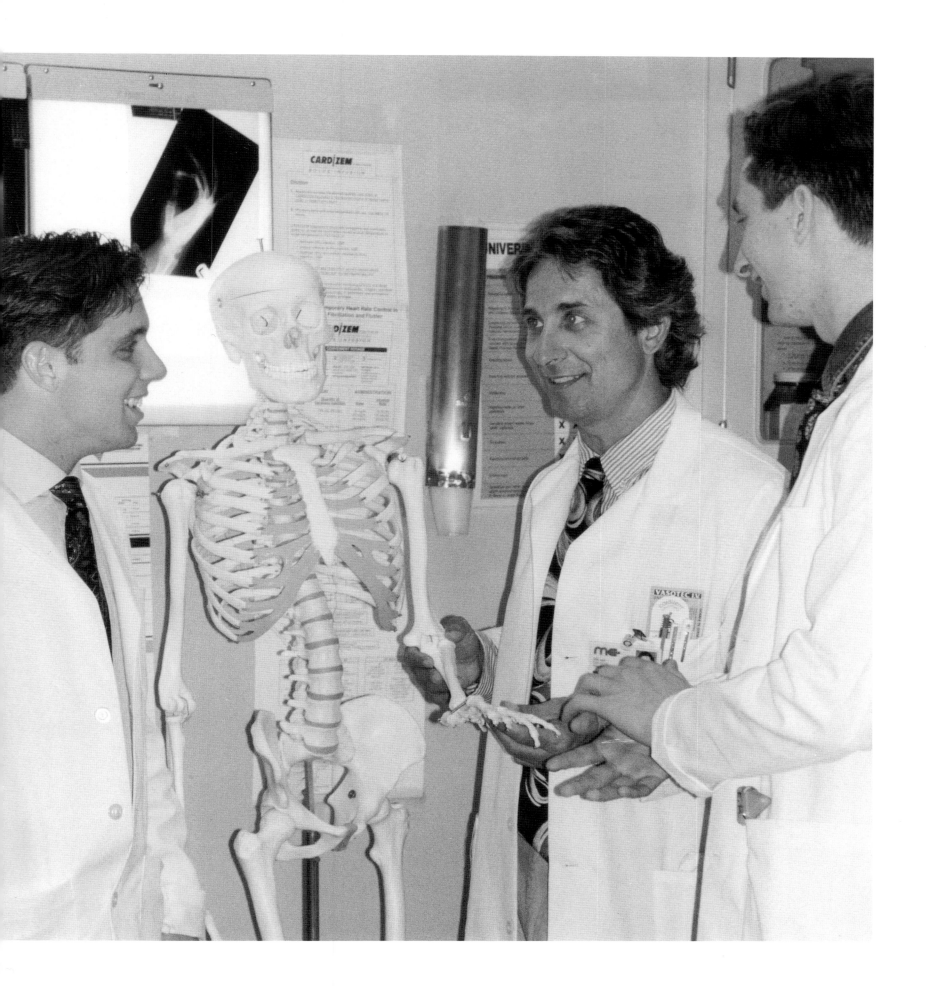

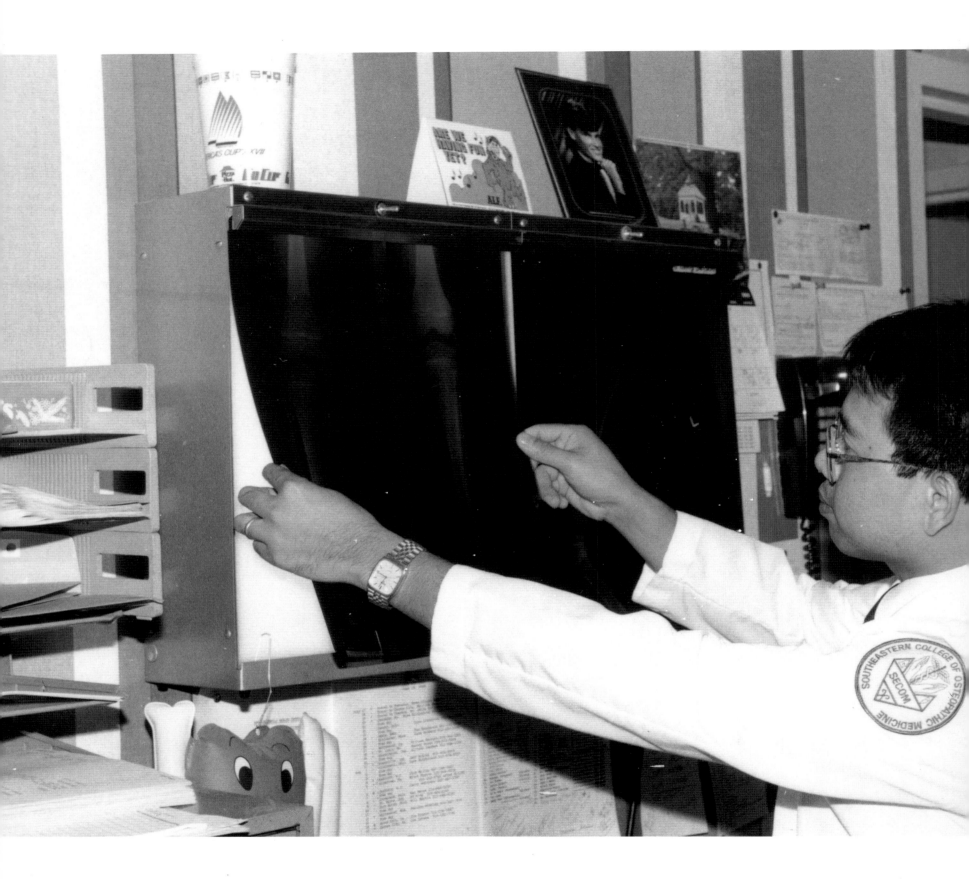

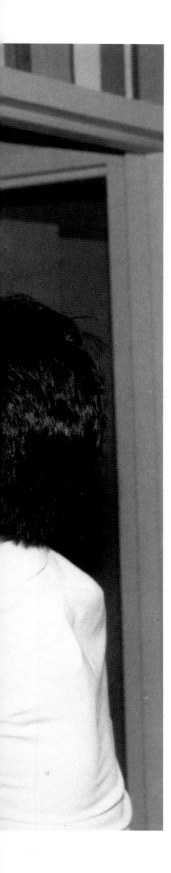

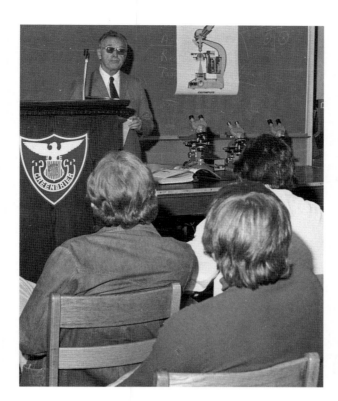 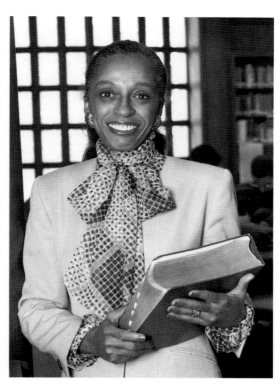

Left: *Students spend two years of their education caring for patients in hospital-based centers and in campus-based clinics, such as this one in Florida.*

Above left: *In the ten years beginning in 1968, the number of osteopathic medical schools increased from five to 14. The West Virginia College of Osteopathic Medicine was founded in 1974 on the site of a former military academy.*

Above right: *From the very first class, women have been welcomed into the osteopathic medical schools. Today, Barbara Ross-Lee, DO, dean at the College of Osteopathic Medicine at Ohio University, is one of thousands of women physicians contributing to the field as educators and/or as practitioners.*

In a variety of venues, osteopathic students continue the tradition of teaching and sharing their knowledge by devoting time to a younger generation.

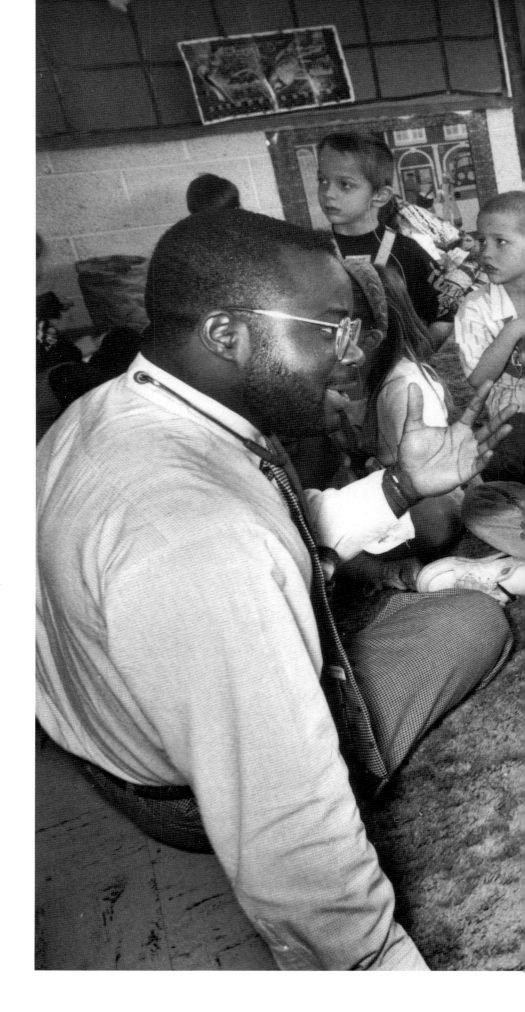

The Ohio School Visit Program sends medical students to public school classroom to demonstrate that it is never too early to learn about good health.

148

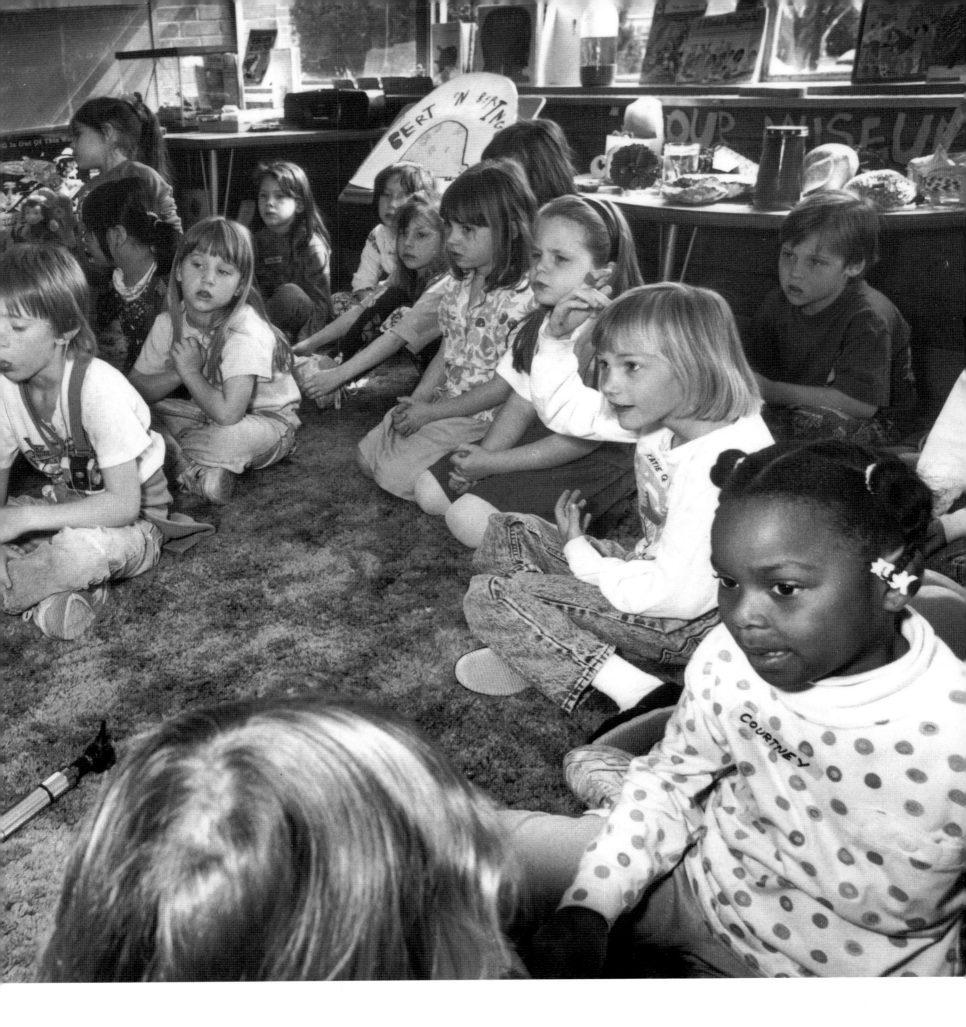

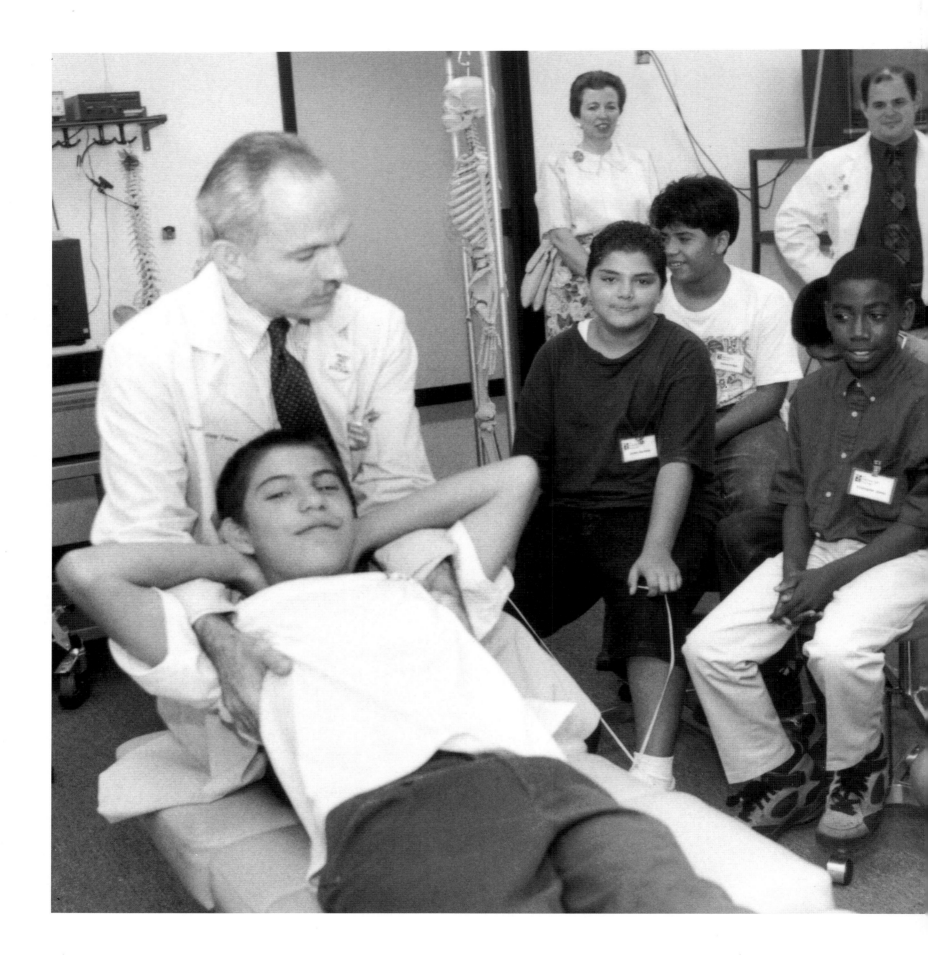

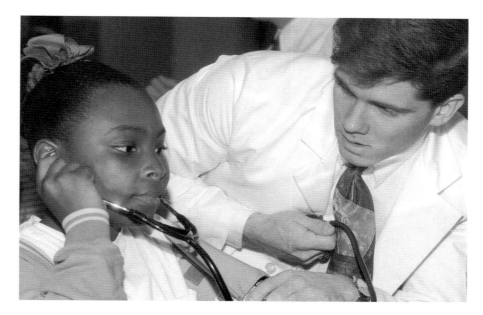

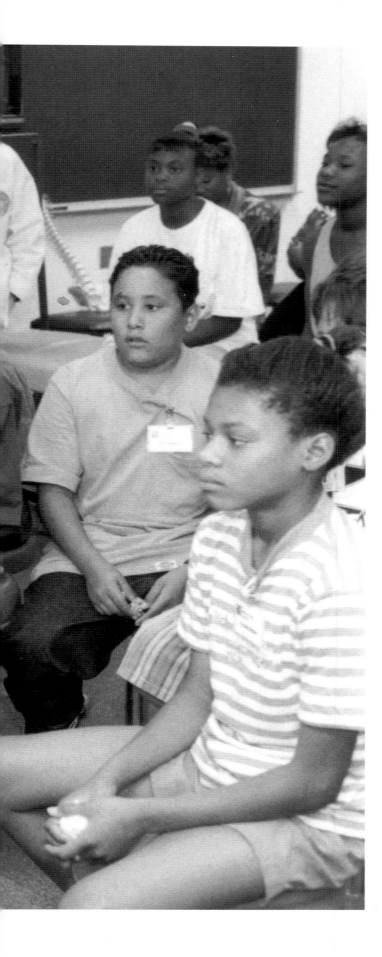

Left: *The osteopathic medical colleges take seriously their role to teach not only the enrolled students but also the communities at large about osteopathic medicine. These middle school students watch a demonstration of osteopathic manipulative therapy during a visit to the University of North Texas campus.*

Above: *A University of North Texas osteopathic student helps an elementary school child listen to her heart beat during a health fair.*

Photo credits

A. T. Still Memorial Library at Kirksville College of Osteopathic Medicine, Kirksville, Missouri—Cover, 10, 11, 12, 13, 14, 16, 17, 18, 19, 20, 21, 22, 23, 24, 25, 26, 27, 28-29, 30, 31, 32, 33, 34, 35, 38, 39, 40-41, 42, 43, 44-45, 46-47, 48, 49, 50, 51, 52, 53, 54, 55, 56-57, 58, 59, 60-61, 62, 63, 66, 70, 73, 74-75, 84, 85, 91, 112, 113, 114-115, 116, 117, 118, 120, 123, 124-125, 126, 127, 128

Chicago Osteopathic Hospitals and Medical Centers, Chicago, Illinois—74, 96

College of Osteopathic Medicine of the Pacific, Pomona, California—89, 106 top

Lake Erie College of Osteopathic Medicine, Erie, Pennsylvania—141, 144-145

Michigan State University, College of Osteopathic Medicine, East Lansing, Michigan—88, 99, 105, 109, 125, 139

National Library of Medicine—64

New York College of Osteopathic Medicine, Old Westbury, New York—93, 100, 101, 122, 130, 136-137

Nova Southeastern University, College of Osteopathic Medicine, North Miami Beach, Florida—106 bottom, 131, 142, 146

Ohio University, College of Osteopathic Medicine, Athens, Ohio—107, 108, 140, 144, 147 right, 148-149

Otto Hagel—76, 77, 78-79

Philadelphia College of Osteopathic Medicine, Philadelphia, Pennsylvania—90, 97, 128-129, 133, 134-135

Still National Osteopathic Museum, Kirksville, Missouri—15, 65 [82.699.01], 67, 68-69, 70-71, 71, 72-73, 73, 80-81

University of New England, College of Osteopathic Medicine, Biddeford, Maine—86-87

University of North Texas, Health Science Center at Fort Worth, Fort Worth, Texas—98 bottom, 103, 120-121, 150-151, 151

University of Osteopathic Medicine, Kansas City, Missouri—132

West Virginia School of Osteopathic Medicine, Lewisburg, West Virginia—86, 92, 94, 98 top, 102, 104, 119, 138-139, 143, 147 left

Bibliography

1. Auxiliary to the AOA Staff. *Still Gathering: A Centennial Celebration*. Chicago, Ill: 1992.

2. Booth ER. *History of Osteopathy and Twentieth Century Medical Practice*. 2nd ed. Cincinnati, Ohio: Caxton Press; 1924.

3. Gevitz N. *The D.O.'s: Osteopathic Medicine in America*. Baltimore, Md: The Johns Hopkins University Press; 1991.

4. Hildreth AG. *The Lengthening Shadow of Andrew Taylor Still*. Kirksville, Mo: Journal Printing; 1942.

5. Keesecker RP, ed. *The Osteopathic Movement in Medicine: A Source Document on the Origin, Growth, and Development of Osteopathy and the Osteopathic Profession*. Chicago, Ill: American Osteopathic Association; 1957.

6. Northup GW. *Osteopathic Medicine: An American Reformation*. Chicago, Ill: American Osteopathic Association; 1966.

7. Northup GW, ed. *Osteopathic Research: Growth and Development*. Chicago, Ill: American Osteopathic Association; 1987.

8. Rothstein WG. *American Physicians in the Nineteenth Century: From Sects to Science*. Baltimore, Md: The Johns Hopkins University Press; 1972.

9. Schnucker RV, ed. *Early Osteopathy in the Words of A.T. Still*. Kirksville, Mo: Thomas Jefferson University Press; 1991.

10. Seyle J. *History of Osteopathic Research*. Chicago, Ill: American Osteopathic Association; 1951.

11. Still AT. *Autobiography of Andrew Taylor Still with a History of the Discovery and Development of the Science of Osteopathy*. Reprint of 1897 edition. Salem, NH: Ayer; 1972.

12. Still CE Jr. *Frontier Doctor—Medical Pioneer*. Kirksville, Mo: Thomas Jefferson University Press; 1991.

13. Trowbridge C. *Andrew Taylor Still*. Kirksville, Mo: Thomas Jefferson University Press; 1991.

14. Walter GW. *Osteopathic Medicine: Past and Present*. 3rd ed. Kirksville, Mo: Kirksville College of Osteopathic Medicine; 1993.

15. Walter GW. *The First School of Osteopathic Medicine*. Kirksville, Mo: Thomas Jefferson University Press; 1992.